NATURAL APPROACH TO BONE HEALTH

Evidence-Based Strategies for Reversing Osteoporosis and Osteopenia

By

Calvin M. Duncan

All rights reserved. No part of this publication may be reproduced, distributed, or transmitted in any form or by any means, including photocopying, recording or other electronic or mechanical methods, without the prior written permission of the publisher, except in the case of brief quotation embodied in critical reviews and certain other noncommercial uses permitted by copyright law

Copyright by Calvin M. Duncan 2023

TABLE OF CONTENTS

INTRODUCTION

Maintaining optimal bone health is crucial for overall well-being and longevity. Bones provide the structural framework for our bodies, supporting movement, protecting vital organs, and serving as a reservoir for essential minerals. Conditions such as osteoporosis and osteopenia, characterized by weakened and porous bones, can significantly impact one's quality of life. While medications are commonly prescribed to address these issues, a growing body of evidence supports the effectiveness of natural approaches in promoting bone health.

In this exploration of natural interventions for bone health, we will delve into the fundamental principles and practices that contribute to strong and resilient bones. This comprehensive guide aims to empower individuals to take a proactive role in enhancing their skeletal well-being through lifestyle modifications, nutritional choices, and evidence-based strategies.

The Complexity of Bone Health:

Bone health is a critical aspect of overall well-being, providing the structural foundation for our bodies and influencing various physiological functions. The complexity of bone health lies in its dynamic nature, involving a constant process of remodeling and adaptation to internal and external factors. To grasp the intricacies of bone health, it is essential to explore the structural composition of bones, the physiological mechanisms governing bone remodeling, and the multifaceted factors influencing bone density and strength.

Bones are remarkable structures comprised of living tissue, primarily bone tissue, collagen, and minerals. The key minerals include calcium and phosphorus, contributing to the hardness and strength of bones. The matrix of collagen provides flexibility and resilience. The combination of these elements forms a dynamic scaffold that not only supports the body's structure but also serves as a reservoir for minerals essential for various physiological processes.

Bone remodeling is a continuous and tightly regulated process that involves the removal of old or damaged bone tissue (resorption) and the formation of new bone tissue (ossification). Specialized cells, including osteoclasts and osteoblasts, orchestrate this process. Osteoclasts break down bone tissue, releasing minerals into the bloodstream, while osteoblasts synthesize new bone tissue.

This dynamic remodeling process plays a crucial role in maintaining bone strength, repairing micro-damage, and adapting to changing mechanical demands. The delicate balance between bone resorption and formation is influenced by various factors, including hormonal signals, mechanical loading, and nutritional status.

Hormones play a pivotal role in bone health, influencing the activity of osteoclasts and osteoblasts. Parathyroid hormone (PTH) and calcitonin, for example, regulate calcium levels in the blood by modulating bone resorption and formation. Estrogen and testosterone also have significant effects on bone density. The decline in estrogen levels during menopause can lead to accelerated bone loss in women.

Bones respond to mechanical forces through a process known as Wolff's law. Regular weight-bearing activities and mechanical loading stimulate bone formation, enhancing density and strength. Conversely, a lack of mechanical loading, as seen in sedentary lifestyles, can lead to bone loss. This highlights the importance of weight-bearing exercises in promoting bone health.

Nutrition plays a critical role in bone health, with calcium and vitamin D being particularly vital. Calcium is a primary component of bone mineral, and adequate intake is necessary for maintaining bone density. Vitamin D facilitates calcium absorption and regulates calcium metabolism. Insufficient levels of these nutrients can compromise bone health and contribute to conditions like osteoporosis.

Beyond structural, hormonal, mechanical, and nutritional aspects, various factors contribute to the complexity of bone health. Genetic predispositions, chronic medical conditions, medications, and lifestyle factors such as smoking and excessive alcohol consumption can impact bone density and fracture risk.

The complexity of bone health stems from the intricate interplay of structural, physiological, hormonal, mechanical, and nutritional factors. Understanding this complexity is essential for developing comprehensive strategies to promote and maintain optimal bone health throughout life. By recognizing the dynamic nature of bones and the various influences on their remodeling, individuals can make informed lifestyle choices to support strong and resilient skeletal structures.

The Limitations of Medication:

The use of medication in addressing bone health issues, such as osteoporosis and osteopenia, has become a common practice in contemporary medicine. While pharmaceutical interventions have demonstrated efficacy in managing these conditions, it is crucial to recognize the limitations associated with long-term medication use and to consider alternative approaches for maintaining and improving bone health.

Before delving into the limitations, it's essential to understand the types of medications commonly prescribed for bone health. Bisphosphonates, such as alendronate and risedronate, are among the most prescribed drugs. They work by inhibiting bone resorption, thereby increasing bone density. Other medications, like hormone therapy and selective estrogen receptor modulators (SERMs), aim to balance hormonal levels, especially in postmenopausal women. Additionally, denosumab, a monoclonal antibody, is used to prevent bone loss.

One of the primary limitations of medication for bone health lies in the potential side effects and associated risks. Bisphosphonates, for example, have been linked to gastrointestinal issues,

musculoskeletal pain, and, in rare cases, osteonecrosis of the jaw. Long-term use of these medications has raised concerns about atypical fractures of the femur. Hormone therapies, particularly in postmenopausal women, may increase the risk of cardiovascular events, stroke, and breast cancer.

The decision to use medication for bone health must be carefully weighed against these potential risks, especially when considering prolonged treatment. Patient-specific factors, including age, overall health, and the presence of other medical conditions, must be taken into account in the risk-benefit analysis.

While medication can slow down bone loss and, in some cases, increase bone density, it often has limited ability to reverse existing damage. Once bones have become porous and weakened, the restoration of their original strength may be challenging. This limitation underscores the importance of early intervention and preventive measures in maintaining optimal bone health.

The long-term use of bone health medications may create a sense of dependency, where individuals rely solely on pharmaceutical interventions without addressing underlying lifestyle factors. A holistic approach to bone health involves not only medication but also lifestyle modifications, nutrition, and physical activity. Depending solely on medication may neglect these crucial components.

Access to bone health medications can be restricted by financial considerations. These medications may be expensive, and not all individuals have adequate insurance coverage. Limited access to medication can impact the continuity of treatment, potentially leading to suboptimal outcomes in bone health.

Adherence to medication regimens is essential for their effectiveness. However, patients may struggle with compliance due to factors such as forgetfulness, side effects, or a reluctance to take medication long-term. Poor adherence can compromise the intended benefits of the treatment.

Responses to medication can vary among individuals. Some may experience significant improvements in bone density and reduced fracture risk, while others may not respond as favorably. This variability underscores the need for personalized approaches to bone health that consider individual characteristics and responses.

Given the limitations associated with medication, there is growing interest in exploring alternative and complementary approaches to bone health. Lifestyle modifications, including a balanced diet rich in essential nutrients, weight-bearing exercises, and stress management, play a crucial role in supporting bone health. Integrative approaches that combine conventional medicine with complementary therapies are gaining attention as a more comprehensive strategy.

While medications have a place in managing bone health issues, it is essential to recognize their limitations. Potential side effects, limited reversibility of bone damage, dependency concerns, cost considerations, patient compliance issues, and individual variability in response all contribute to the complex landscape of medication use for bone health. A holistic approach that includes lifestyle modifications and considers individual needs may offer a more comprehensive and sustainable approach to maintaining and improving bone health over the long term.

The Rise of Natural Approaches:

The rise of natural approaches in addressing and promoting bone health reflects a growing recognition of the limitations and potential drawbacks associated with traditional pharmaceutical interventions. As individuals seek alternatives that prioritize holistic well-being and minimize the impact of side effects, natural approaches have gained prominence in the field of bone health. These approaches encompass a wide range of lifestyle modifications, dietary strategies, and evidence-based practices aimed at enhancing bone density and strength.

Natural approaches to bone health are rooted in a holistic perspective that considers the interconnectedness of various factors influencing skeletal well-being. Unlike the targeted nature of pharmaceutical interventions, which often focus on inhibiting bone resorption or modifying hormonal levels, natural approaches take into account the broader context of an individual's lifestyle, nutrition, and overall health.

One fundamental pillar of natural approaches to bone health is the incorporation of lifestyle modifications. Regular weight-bearing exercises, such as walking, jogging, and resistance training, play a crucial role in stimulating bone formation and maintaining bone density. Engaging in physical activities that subject bones to mechanical loading promotes skeletal strength and resilience.

Furthermore, avoiding sedentary behavior is essential, as prolonged periods of inactivity can contribute to bone loss. Incorporating movement into daily routines and adopting an active lifestyle contribute to overall well-being and support bone health.

Nutrition is a cornerstone of natural approaches to bone health. Adequate intake of essential nutrients, particularly calcium and vitamin D, is crucial for maintaining bone density. Calcium is a key mineral in bone composition, and insufficient levels can lead to weakened bones. Vitamin D facilitates calcium absorption and is essential for bone health.

In addition to these key nutrients, a well-balanced diet that includes a variety of vitamins and minerals contributes to overall health, indirectly benefiting bone health. Nutrient-rich foods, such as fruits, vegetables, whole grains, and lean proteins, provide the necessary building blocks for strong and resilient bones.

While natural approaches acknowledge the importance of hormonal balance, they focus on lifestyle practices that naturally support hormonal health. Adequate sleep, for example, plays a crucial role in hormonal regulation, including the release of growth hormone, which contributes to bone density. Stress management techniques, such as meditation and yoga, can help regulate cortisol levels, preventing excessive bone resorption.

The rise of natural approaches has also led to increased interest in integrative therapies that complement conventional strategies. Complementary practices such as acupuncture and herbal medicine are being explored for their potential benefits in bone health. While more research is needed to establish the efficacy of these approaches, their inclusion in the conversation reflects a broader shift towards personalized and comprehensive care.

Natural approaches aim to address underlying causes of bone health issues rather than merely managing symptoms. This involves identifying and addressing factors such as nutritional deficiencies, hormonal imbalances, and lifestyle habits that contribute to bone loss. By targeting these root causes, natural approaches seek to create a foundation for sustained and long-term improvements in bone health.

A notable aspect of the rise of natural approaches in bone health is the emphasis on patient empowerment. Individuals are encouraged to take an active role in their well-being by making informed choices about their lifestyle, nutrition, and overall health. This proactive approach aligns with the principles of preventive medicine and fosters a sense of agency in maintaining and improving bone health.

While the shift towards natural approaches is driven by a desire for holistic care, it is essential to highlight that these strategies are grounded in scientific evidence. Research studies continue to explore the effectiveness of natural interventions in improving bone health, providing a solid foundation for the integration of these approaches into mainstream care.

Despite the growing popularity of natural approaches, challenges and considerations exist. The lack of standardization in some complementary therapies, varying individual responses, and the need for further research are important aspects to acknowledge. Integrating natural approaches into mainstream healthcare requires a collaborative effort involving healthcare professionals, researchers, and individuals seeking alternative solutions.

The rise of natural approaches in bone health reflects a paradigm shift towards holistic and patient-centered care. By embracing lifestyle modifications, nutritional strategies, and integrative therapies, individuals are exploring alternatives that prioritize overall well-being and minimize the potential drawbacks associated with traditional medications. The evidence-based nature of these approaches, combined with a focus on addressing underlying causes and empowering individuals, positions natural interventions as valuable components in the comprehensive care of bone health. As research continues to unfold, the integration of natural approaches into mainstream healthcare holds promise for a more personalized and effective approach to maintaining and improving bone health.

Empowering Individuals:

Empowering individuals to take an active and informed role in their bone health is a crucial aspect of the paradigm shift towards natural approaches. In the context of promoting skeletal well-being through lifestyle modifications, nutritional choices, and evidence-based practices, empowerment involves fostering a sense of agency, providing education, and encouraging proactive engagement. By empowering individuals, the aim is to create a foundation for sustained and personalized efforts that contribute to strong and resilient bones throughout life.

Central to empowering individuals for a natural approach to bone health is education. Understanding the basic principles of bone physiology, the impact of lifestyle choices, and the role

of nutrition is foundational. Education equips individuals with the knowledge needed to make informed decisions about their bone health, allowing them to navigate the complexities of natural approaches with confidence.

Educational initiatives can take various forms, including public health campaigns, community workshops, and online resources. These platforms serve to disseminate information about the importance of bone health, the interplay of various factors, and the potential benefits of natural interventions. By raising awareness and providing accessible information, education becomes a catalyst for proactive engagement.

Empowering individuals for a natural approach to bone health involves fostering a proactive mindset. This mindset encourages individuals to view bone health as a dynamic aspect of their overall well-being that requires continuous attention and care. Rather than reactive responses to bone-related issues, a proactive mindset emphasizes preventive measures and lifestyle choices that contribute to long-term skeletal health.

Encouraging individuals to adopt a proactive mindset involves shifting the narrative from a focus on treating existing conditions to preventing future challenges. This change in perspective positions individuals as active participants in their health journey, motivating them to make choices that support and enhance their bone health throughout different stages of life.

Empowerment in the context of bone health recognizes the diversity of individuals and the need for personalized approaches. One size does not fit all, and empowering individuals involves tailoring recommendations to their unique circumstances, including age, gender, genetics, and existing health conditions. Personalized approaches acknowledge that each person's journey to optimal bone health is distinct and may require different strategies.

This emphasis on personalization extends to the integration of natural approaches into an individual's lifestyle. For example, a personalized exercise plan may take into account a person's fitness level, preferences, and any existing musculoskeletal conditions. Similarly, nutritional recommendations may be customized based on dietary preferences, cultural factors, and specific nutrient needs.

Empowering individuals for a natural approach to bone health also involves building self-efficacy, which is the belief in one's ability to take meaningful action and produce desired outcomes. This psychological concept is crucial in fostering a sense of control and confidence in managing one's bone health. Building self-efficacy requires a combination of education, support, and positive reinforcement.

Practical tools, such as goal-setting frameworks and tracking mechanisms, can contribute to building self-efficacy. For instance, setting achievable goals related to regular physical activity, dietary choices, and other lifestyle modifications allows individuals to experience a sense of accomplishment, reinforcing their belief in their ability to positively impact their bone health.

In the digital age, technology plays a significant role in empowering individuals for a natural approach to bone health. Mobile applications, wearable devices, and online platforms provide accessible tools for tracking physical activity, monitoring nutritional intake, and receiving

personalized health information. These technologies can enhance engagement, provide real-time feedback, and serve as valuable resources for individuals seeking to prioritize their bone health.

The use of technology also facilitates remote access to educational materials, virtual consultations with healthcare professionals, and online communities where individuals can share experiences and support each other. By leveraging technology, empowerment becomes more accessible and adaptable to the diverse needs of individuals.

Empowering individuals for a natural approach to bone health requires communication that is inclusive, culturally sensitive, and easily understandable. Information should be presented in a way that resonates with diverse audiences, considering linguistic differences, cultural beliefs, and varying levels of health literacy. Inclusive communication ensures that individuals from different backgrounds feel acknowledged and included in the conversation about bone health.

Additionally, open and non-judgmental communication is essential in empowering individuals to make informed choices without feeling overwhelmed or stigmatized. Creating a supportive environment where questions are welcomed, concerns are addressed, and progress is celebrated fosters a culture of empowerment and collaboration.

Empowerment extends beyond individual efforts and encompasses community engagement and support. Creating a supportive community where individuals can share experiences, exchange information, and offer encouragement contributes to a collective sense of empowerment.

Community-based initiatives, such as local fitness groups, cooking classes, or bone health awareness campaigns, provide opportunities for individuals to connect with like-minded peers and reinforce their commitment to natural approaches.

Peer support and shared experiences can be powerful motivators, fostering a sense of belonging and shared responsibility for bone health. Additionally, community-based programs can leverage local resources and cultural contexts to make empowerment initiatives more relevant and impactful.

Recognizing and addressing potential barriers to empowerment is a crucial aspect of promoting natural approaches to bone health. Economic constraints, limited access to healthcare resources, cultural factors, and competing priorities can pose challenges for individuals seeking to prioritize their bone health. Empowerment initiatives should aim to identify and address these barriers through targeted interventions, community partnerships, and advocacy efforts.

Overcoming barriers also involves acknowledging the socio-economic determinants that can influence an individual's ability to engage in natural approaches. By addressing systemic issues related to healthcare access, education, and social support, empowerment initiatives can contribute to creating more equitable opportunities for individuals to prioritize their bone health.

Empowering individuals for a natural approach to bone health is a multifaceted endeavor that involves education, fostering a proactive mindset, personalization, building self-efficacy, leveraging technology, inclusive communication, community engagement, and overcoming barriers. This empowerment goes beyond merely providing information; it involves creating a

supportive environment where individuals feel capable, motivated, and connected in their journey towards optimal bone health.

As the paradigm shifts towards holistic and patient-centered care, the role of empowerment becomes increasingly pivotal. Individuals armed with knowledge, a sense of agency, and a supportive community are better equipped to navigate the complexities of natural approaches to bone health. By fostering empowerment, the goal is to inspire a proactive and sustained commitment to lifestyle modifications, nutritional choices, and evidence-based practices that contribute to strong and resilient bones throughout life.

In the following sections, we will explore the multifaceted aspects of natural approaches to bone health. From understanding the impact of nutrition and exercise on bone density to delving into the role of hormones and stress, each chapter will provide valuable insights and practical tips. By the end of this guide, readers will be equipped with a comprehensive understanding of how natural interventions can be incorporated into their lives to foster strong and resilient bones.

CHAPTER ONE
Understanding Osteoporosis and Osteopenia

Osteoporosis:

Osteoporosis is a systemic skeletal disorder characterized by low bone mass and microarchitectural deterioration of bone tissue, leading to an increased risk of fractures. This condition has far-reaching implications for individuals' health and well-being, often resulting in pain, reduced mobility, and a significant impact on the quality of life. In this comprehensive exploration, we will delve into the intricate details of osteoporosis, including its pathophysiology, risk factors, clinical manifestations, diagnostic methods, and management strategies.

Pathophysiology of Osteoporosis:

Understanding the pathophysiology of osteoporosis is fundamental to unraveling the complexities of this skeletal disorder. The process of bone remodeling, governed by the delicate balance between bone resorption and formation, plays a central role.

a. Bone Remodeling:

Bone remodeling is a continuous and dynamic process crucial for maintaining bone integrity. Specialized cells, osteoclasts, and osteoblasts orchestrate this process. Osteoclasts are responsible for breaking down old or damaged bone tissue, releasing minerals into the bloodstream. Osteoblasts, on the other hand, synthesize new bone tissue, contributing to bone formation.

This constant cycle of resorption and formation ensures that bones remain strong and adapt to changing mechanical demands. However, in osteoporosis, this balance is disrupted, with an increased rate of bone resorption and a decreased rate of bone formation, leading to a net loss of bone mass.

b. Bone Microarchitecture Changes:

In addition to alterations in bone remodeling, osteoporosis is characterized by changes in bone microarchitecture. The trabecular and cortical components of bone undergo structural deterioration, resulting in a porous and weakened bone matrix. The loss of trabecular connectivity and thinning of cortical bone contribute to decreased bone strength and an increased susceptibility to fractures.

Risk Factors for Osteoporosis:

Several factors contribute to the development of osteoporosis, encompassing genetic, hormonal, lifestyle, and nutritional elements. Understanding these risk factors is crucial for identifying individuals who may be more susceptible to bone loss.

a. Genetic Predisposition:

Genetic factors play a significant role in determining an individual's predisposition to osteoporosis. Family history of the condition, especially a history of fractures in parents or siblings, may increase the likelihood of developing osteoporosis. Genetic variations influencing bone density and structure contribute to the hereditary component of this disorder.

b. Hormonal Influences:

Hormonal changes, particularly those associated with menopause in women and aging in both genders, contribute significantly to the development of osteoporosis. Estrogen, a hormone that plays a protective role in bone health, declines during menopause, leading to accelerated bone loss in women. Similarly, a gradual decrease in testosterone levels in men is associated with reduced bone density.

c. Nutritional Deficiencies:

Adequate nutrition is essential for maintaining optimal bone health. Calcium and vitamin D are crucial nutrients for bone formation and maintenance. Inadequate intake of these nutrients can compromise bone density and increase the risk of osteoporosis. Other nutritional factors, including vitamin K, magnesium, and phosphorus, also contribute to bone health.

d. Lifestyle Choices:

Certain lifestyle choices can significantly impact bone health and contribute to the development of osteoporosis. Lack of physical activity, especially weight-bearing exercises, can lead to decreased bone density. Smoking has been linked to reduced bone mass, impaired bone quality, and an increased risk of fractures. Excessive alcohol consumption can interfere with calcium absorption and contribute to bone loss.

e. Medical Conditions and Medications:

Several medical conditions and medications can increase the risk of osteoporosis. Chronic conditions such as rheumatoid arthritis, celiac disease, and hormonal disorders may impact bone density. Long-term use of medications like corticosteroids, commonly prescribed for inflammatory conditions, can contribute to bone loss. It is crucial for healthcare providers to assess the potential impact of underlying medical conditions and medications on bone health.

Clinical Manifestations of Osteoporosis:

Osteoporosis is often asymptomatic until a fracture occurs. Fractures resulting from weakened bones are a hallmark manifestation of this condition, with common sites including the spine, hips, and wrists.

a. Vertebral Fractures:

Vertebral fractures, often termed compression fractures, can lead to a reduction in height and a stooped or hunched posture. These fractures may cause chronic back pain, decreased mobility, and limitations in performing daily activities. Multiple vertebral fractures can result in significant deformities and adversely affect an individual's quality of life.

b. Hip Fractures:

Hip fractures are particularly severe and are associated with increased mortality and a significant decline in functional independence. Recovery from a hip fracture often involves surgical intervention, rehabilitation, and long-term care. The consequences of hip fractures extend beyond the physical aspects and may lead to emotional and psychological challenges.

c. Wrist and Forearm Fractures:

Fractures in the wrist and forearm can impact an individual's ability to perform routine tasks and may necessitate adaptations in daily activities. These fractures often occur as a result of falls or trauma and can be a warning sign of compromised bone health.

Diagnostic Methods for Osteoporosis:

Early detection of osteoporosis is crucial for implementing preventive measures and minimizing the risk of fractures. Several diagnostic methods are employed to assess bone density and evaluate an individual's fracture risk.

a. Dual-Energy X-ray Absorptiometry (DXA):

DXA scans are the gold standard for measuring bone mineral density (BMD) and are widely used for diagnosing osteoporosis. These scans involve low levels of radiation and are typically performed at the hip and spine. The results are reported as a T-score, which compares an individual's BMD to that of a healthy young adult. A T-score of -2.5 or lower is indicative of osteoporosis.

b. Quantitative Ultrasound (QUS):

Quantitative ultrasound is an alternative method for assessing bone density, particularly at peripheral sites such as the heel or finger. While not as widely used as DXA, QUS provides additional information about bone quality and may be utilized in specific clinical settings.

c. Laboratory Tests:

Blood tests may be conducted to assess hormonal levels and rule out underlying medical conditions contributing to bone loss. These tests include measurements of calcium, vitamin D, parathyroid hormone (PTH), and markers of bone turnover.

d. Clinical Evaluation:

A thorough medical history, including family history, and a physical examination are integral components of the diagnostic process. Evaluating risk factors, assessing lifestyle choices, and identifying signs of previous fractures contribute to a comprehensive understanding of an individual's bone health.

Management Strategies for Osteoporosis:

Managing osteoporosis involves a multifaceted approach aimed at optimizing bone health, preventing fractures, and addressing underlying causes.

a. Pharmacological Interventions:

Pharmacological interventions are often prescribed to manage osteoporosis and prevent further bone loss. Bisphosphonates, such as alendronate and risedronate, are commonly prescribed to inhibit bone resorption and increase bone density. Other medications, including selective estrogen receptor modulators (SERMs), hormone therapy, and denosumab, may also be considered based on individual risk factors and preferences.

b. Calcium and Vitamin D Supplementation:

Adequate intake of calcium and vitamin D is essential for maintaining bone health. Calcium supplements may be recommended for individuals with insufficient dietary intake, especially those at risk of deficiency. Vitamin D supplementation is often prescribed, particularly in individuals with limited sun exposure, as vitamin D facilitates calcium absorption.

c. Lifestyle Modifications:

Incorporating lifestyle modifications is integral to managing osteoporosis. Weight-bearing exercises, such as walking, jogging, and resistance training, stimulate bone formation and improve overall bone health. Smoking cessation is encouraged, as smoking has detrimental effects on bone density. Limiting alcohol intake and maintaining a balanced diet rich in essential nutrients contribute to holistic bone health.

d. Fall Prevention Strategies:

Fall prevention is a crucial aspect of managing osteoporosis, especially in older individuals who may be at an increased risk of fractures. Home safety assessments, balance exercises, and addressing factors contributing to falls can significantly reduce the risk of fractures.

e. Patient Education and Support:

Patient education plays a pivotal role in managing osteoporosis. Individuals should be informed about the importance of adherence to medications, lifestyle modifications, and regular follow-up appointments. Providing support and addressing concerns about treatment can enhance patient engagement and improve overall outcomes.

f. Monitoring and Follow-Up:

Regular monitoring and follow-up are essential components of osteoporosis management. Periodic DXA scans assess changes in bone density, allowing healthcare providers to adjust treatment plans as needed. Monitoring for potential side effects of medications and addressing any emerging risk factors contribute to ongoing care.

Ongoing Research and Advancements:

Ongoing research and advancements in osteoporosis contribute to a deeper understanding of the condition, paving the way for more effective prevention, diagnosis, and treatment strategies. The dynamic nature of scientific inquiry continues to uncover new insights into the underlying mechanisms of osteoporosis, explore novel therapeutic interventions, and refine approaches to managing bone health.

Advancements in genetic research have illuminated the role of specific genetic factors in influencing bone density and susceptibility to osteoporosis. Researchers are identifying genetic markers associated with bone health, fracture risk, and response to treatments. This knowledge holds the potential for personalized medicine approaches, allowing healthcare providers to tailor interventions based on an individual's genetic profile. Understanding the genetic basis of osteoporosis enables more precise risk assessment and targeted therapeutic strategies.

Emerging therapies specifically target bone metabolism, aiming to modulate the delicate balance between bone resorption and formation. Anti-resorptive medications, such as monoclonal antibodies and receptor activator of nuclear factor-kappaB ligand (RANKL) inhibitors, are designed to inhibit osteoclast activity, thereby reducing bone resorption. Anabolic agents, such as parathyroid hormone analogs, stimulate bone formation. Ongoing research explores the safety, efficacy, and long-term outcomes of these bone-targeted therapies, with a focus on optimizing their use for various patient populations.

Advancements in imaging technologies contribute to more accurate assessments of bone density and microarchitecture. High-resolution imaging techniques, such as high-resolution peripheral quantitative computed tomography (HR-pQCT), provide detailed three-dimensional images of bone structure. These techniques offer valuable insights into trabecular and cortical bone compartments, aiding in the early detection of changes associated with osteoporosis. Improved imaging technologies enhance diagnostic precision and enable monitoring of treatment efficacy.

Biomarkers that reflect bone turnover are under investigation for their utility in assessing bone health and response to treatment. These biomarkers include specific molecules released during bone resorption and formation processes. Monitoring changes in these biomarkers may offer insights into the dynamic aspects of bone metabolism, allowing for early identification of individuals at risk of osteoporosis and facilitating personalized treatment plans.

Research continues to explore the role of nutrition in maintaining optimal bone health. Studies investigate the impact of various nutrients, including calcium, vitamin D, vitamin K, magnesium, and others, on bone density and fracture risk. Understanding the intricate relationship between nutrition and bone health informs dietary recommendations and supplementation strategies. Additionally, research explores the potential benefits of bioactive compounds, such as phytoestrogens and polyphenols, in supporting bone health.

Ongoing research emphasizes the importance of physical activity in promoting bone health. Studies explore the specific types, intensity, and duration of exercises that optimize bone density and strength. Tailoring exercise interventions to individual needs and preferences is a focus of ongoing research. Understanding the molecular mechanisms through which exercise influences bone remodeling provides valuable insights into the development of targeted exercise prescriptions for individuals at risk of osteoporosis.

Advancements in digital health technologies and telemedicine enhance the delivery of osteoporosis care. Mobile applications and wearable devices facilitate remote monitoring of physical activity, medication adherence, and lifestyle factors that impact bone health. Telemedicine platforms enable virtual consultations, improving accessibility to healthcare services, especially for individuals in remote or underserved areas. Integrating digital health tools into osteoporosis management enhances patient engagement and supports long-term adherence to treatment plans.

Sophisticated tools for assessing fracture risk are continually evolving. Fracture risk assessment algorithms incorporate a combination of clinical risk factors, bone mineral density measurements, and, in some cases, genetic information. Ongoing research refines these tools to enhance their accuracy and applicability across diverse populations. Improved risk stratification contributes to more targeted interventions and resource allocation for fracture prevention.

While postmenopausal women have traditionally been the focus of hormonal therapies for osteoporosis, ongoing research explores the impact of hormonal interventions in men. Testosterone replacement therapy and selective estrogen receptor modulators (SERMs) are being investigated for their efficacy in preserving bone density and reducing fracture risk in men with age-related bone loss. Understanding the hormonal influences on bone health in both genders contributes to more inclusive and effective treatment strategies.

Patient-centered outcomes research emphasizes the incorporation of patient perspectives and preferences into osteoporosis care. Studies assess the impact of osteoporosis and its treatments on patients' quality of life, adherence to medications, and satisfaction with care. This patient-centric approach informs the development of interventions that align with individuals' values and priorities, fostering greater engagement in bone health management.

In conclusion, ongoing research and advancements in osteoporosis underscore the dynamic nature of scientific inquiry in the field of bone health. The convergence of genetic insights, innovative therapies, advanced imaging technologies, and patient-centered research holds promise for more effective preventive strategies, personalized treatment approaches, and improved outcomes for individuals affected by osteoporosis. As the landscape of osteoporosis research continues to evolve, the goal remains to translate scientific discoveries into tangible benefits for individuals at risk of or living with this prevalent skeletal disorder.

Public Health Implications:

The public health implications of osteoporosis are significant, considering its prevalence, impact on healthcare resources, and the potential for disability and mortality associated with fractures. Osteoporosis poses challenges on both individual and societal levels, necessitating public health initiatives focused on education, prevention, and early detection. Addressing the public health implications of osteoporosis involves a multifaceted approach to reduce the burden of this skeletal disorder.

Osteoporosis is a widespread health concern, particularly as populations age. The prevalence of osteoporosis and low bone mass is substantial, affecting millions of individuals worldwide. As life expectancy increases, the number of people at risk for osteoporosis-related fractures is expected to rise, contributing to the overall economic burden on healthcare systems.

Fractures resulting from osteoporosis, especially hip fractures, often require hospitalization, surgery, and rehabilitation. The associated healthcare costs, including medical interventions, medications, and long-term care, place a strain on healthcare resources. Public health initiatives must address the economic impact of osteoporosis to ensure the sustainability of healthcare systems.

Osteoporosis-related fractures can lead to significant disability and a diminished quality of life. Vertebral fractures, in particular, may result in chronic back pain, reduced mobility, and limitations in performing daily activities. Hip fractures, with their associated morbidity and mortality, can lead to long-term disability and a decline in functional independence.

The impact on quality of life extends beyond the physical consequences. Individuals with osteoporosis may experience emotional and psychological distress due to the fear of fractures, pain, and limitations in daily activities. Addressing the public health implications of osteoporosis requires strategies that not only focus on reducing fractures but also on improving the overall well-being of affected individuals.

Given that falls are a major contributor to osteoporosis-related fractures, public health initiatives should prioritize fall prevention programs. These programs aim to reduce the risk of falls, especially among older adults who may be more susceptible to fractures. Fall prevention strategies include educational campaigns, environmental modifications, exercise programs to improve balance and strength, and regular assessments of individuals' risk factors for falls.

By implementing comprehensive fall prevention initiatives, public health efforts can play a crucial role in reducing the incidence of fractures associated with osteoporosis, thereby mitigating the associated disability and healthcare costs.

Public health initiatives should prioritize education and awareness campaigns to increase knowledge about osteoporosis, its risk factors, and preventive measures. Raising awareness among healthcare professionals, individuals at risk, and the general public is essential for early detection and intervention.

Educational campaigns can emphasize the importance of a healthy lifestyle, including adequate calcium and vitamin D intake, regular physical activity, and strategies to prevent falls. Targeted messaging can help dispel myths and misconceptions surrounding osteoporosis, encouraging individuals to proactively manage their bone health.

Public health efforts should promote screening and early detection of osteoporosis, particularly in high-risk populations. Dual-energy X-ray absorptiometry (DXA) scans, which measure bone mineral density, are valuable tools for assessing fracture risk. Outreach programs and collaborations with healthcare providers can facilitate access to screening, ensuring that individuals at risk receive timely assessments.

By promoting routine bone health assessments and integrating osteoporosis screening into regular healthcare check-ups, public health initiatives can contribute to early intervention and the prevention of fractures.

Advocating for policies that support bone health and osteoporosis prevention is a crucial aspect of public health efforts. This includes promoting policies that ensure access to preventive measures, such as nutritional supplements, physical activity programs, and screening services. Additionally, policies that address environmental factors contributing to falls, such as infrastructure modifications in public spaces, can play a role in preventing fractures.

Public health advocacy can also involve supporting research initiatives, promoting evidence-based guidelines for osteoporosis management, and collaborating with policymakers to integrate bone health considerations into broader public health strategies.

Engaging communities in osteoporosis awareness and prevention is vital for the success of public health initiatives. Community-based programs, workshops, and support groups can provide valuable resources and foster a sense of collective responsibility for bone health.

Community engagement initiatives can be tailored to the specific needs and cultural contexts of diverse populations, ensuring that educational materials and interventions are accessible and resonate with different communities. Peer support and shared experiences within communities can contribute to a culture of proactive bone health management.

Public health efforts should prioritize addressing health disparities related to osteoporosis. Certain populations, including women, older adults, and individuals with lower socio-economic status, may face higher risks of osteoporosis and fractures. Culturally competent and inclusive strategies should be developed to reach and serve these populations effectively. Addressing health disparities may involve targeted outreach programs, community partnerships, and policies that aim to reduce barriers to access preventive measures and healthcare services.

Effective public health initiatives necessitate collaboration with healthcare providers. By working in tandem with primary care physicians, specialists, and other healthcare professionals, public health efforts can ensure a continuum of care for individuals at risk of osteoporosis.

This collaboration includes facilitating education and training for healthcare professionals on osteoporosis management, promoting bone health assessments during routine healthcare visits, and fostering communication between public health agencies and healthcare providers.

Public health strategies for osteoporosis should be informed by ongoing research and surveillance efforts. Surveillance systems can monitor trends in osteoporosis prevalence, fracture rates, and the effectiveness of preventive measures. Research initiatives can explore innovative approaches to osteoporosis prevention, such as personalized medicine, advancements in bone-targeted therapies, and the impact of lifestyle interventions. By staying informed about the evolving landscape of osteoporosis research, public health initiatives can adapt and refine their strategies to reflect the latest evidence-based practices.

Addressing the public health implications of osteoporosis requires a comprehensive and collaborative approach that spans education, prevention, early detection, policy advocacy, community engagement, and ongoing research. By prioritizing bone health at

In conclusion, osteoporosis is a complex skeletal disorder with profound implications for individuals' health and well-being. Understanding its pathophysiology, risk factors, clinical manifestations, diagnostic methods, and management strategies is essential for healthcare providers, individuals at risk, and the broader community. By adopting a comprehensive and multidisciplinary approach, including pharmacological interventions, lifestyle modifications, and ongoing monitoring, it is possible to optimize bone health, prevent fractures, and improve the overall quality of life for individuals affected by osteoporosis. Ongoing research and advancements in the field offer hope for more targeted and personalized approaches in the future, further enhancing our ability to address this prevalent and impactful condition.

Osteopenia:

Osteopenia is a term used to describe a condition characterized by lower than normal bone mineral density (BMD) but not to the extent seen in osteoporosis. It represents an intermediate stage between normal bone density and osteoporosis, signaling that bone density is lower than optimal but not yet at a level where the risk of fractures is significantly increased. In this comprehensive exploration, we will delve into the intricacies of osteopenia, including its definition, causes, risk factors, diagnosis, management, and the significance it holds in the broader context of bone health.

Osteopenia is defined by a bone mineral density T-score between -1.0 and -2.5, as measured by dual-energy X-ray absorptiometry (DXA). The T-score compares an individual's bone density to that of a healthy young adult, with a T-score of -1.0 to -2.5 indicating lower bone density than the young adult reference. While osteopenia is not a disease in itself, it serves as an important indicator of compromised bone health and an increased risk of developing osteoporosis.

Understanding the clinical significance of osteopenia involves recognizing its role as a precursor to osteoporosis. Individuals with osteopenia have a bone density that is below the normal range, but the degree of bone loss is not yet at the level observed in osteoporosis. This intermediate stage provides an opportunity for preventive interventions to mitigate further bone loss and reduce the risk of progressing to osteoporosis and associated fractures.

Causes and Risk Factors:

Several factors contribute to the development of osteopenia, and understanding these causes and risk factors is crucial for identifying individuals at risk and implementing preventive measures. Here are the primary causes and risk factors associated with osteopenia:

1. Hormonal Changes:

Hormonal imbalances are significant contributors to the development of osteopenia. Hormones play a crucial role in regulating bone remodeling, which involves the continuous process of bone resorption and formation. Changes in hormonal levels can disrupt this balance, leading to bone loss.

- Estrogen Deficiency: In women, a decline in estrogen levels, particularly during menopause, is a major risk factor for osteopenia. Estrogen has a protective effect on bone density, and its reduction can result in increased bone resorption and decreased bone formation.

- Androgen Deficiency: While estrogen decline is more pronounced in women, men also experience hormonal changes with age. Reduced levels of testosterone in men can contribute to bone loss and the development of osteopenia.

2. Aging:

Advancing age is a natural risk factor for osteopenia. The aging process is associated with changes in bone density and structure. As individuals age, bone remodeling becomes less efficient, leading to a gradual decline in bone mass. The aging-related decline in bone density is not uniform and can be influenced by various factors, including genetics and lifestyle.

3. Genetics:

Genetic factors play a significant role in determining an individual's susceptibility to osteopenia. Specific genetic variations influence bone density, structure, and the rate of bone turnover. Individuals with a family history of osteoporosis or osteopenia may be at an increased risk due to inherited genetic factors.

4. Nutritional Deficiencies:

Adequate nutrition is crucial for maintaining optimal bone health, and deficiencies in certain nutrients can contribute to the development of osteopenia.

- Calcium Deficiency: Calcium is a fundamental mineral for bone formation, and insufficient intake can lead to weakened bones. Chronic calcium deficiency prompts the body to increase bone resorption to maintain calcium homeostasis.

- Vitamin D Deficiency: Vitamin D is essential for calcium absorption and bone mineralization. Insufficient vitamin D levels can impair calcium absorption, negatively impacting bone health.

5. Lifestyle Choices:

Certain lifestyle choices can contribute to the development of osteopenia, either directly or indirectly affecting bone health.

- Physical Inactivity: Lack of regular physical activity, especially weight-bearing exercises, can lead to decreased bone density. Weight-bearing exercises stimulate bone formation and help maintain bone mass.

- Smoking: Smoking has detrimental effects on bone health. It is associated with decreased bone density and an increased risk of fractures. Smoking cessation is an important step in preventing further bone loss.

- Excessive Alcohol Consumption: Excessive alcohol intake is linked to bone loss and an increased risk of fractures. It can interfere with calcium absorption and negatively impact bone density.

6. Medical Conditions:

Certain medical conditions can contribute to osteopenia, either directly through their impact on bone metabolism or indirectly through medications used for treatment.

- Rheumatoid Arthritis: Chronic inflammatory conditions like rheumatoid arthritis can contribute to bone loss. Inflammatory processes affect bone remodeling, leading to increased bone resorption and decreased bone formation.

- Endocrine Disorders: Disorders affecting the endocrine system, such as hyperparathyroidism or hyperthyroidism, can disrupt the hormonal balance involved in bone remodeling.

7. Medications:

Certain medications are known to have adverse effects on bone health and can contribute to the development of osteopenia.

- Glucocorticoids (Steroids): Long-term use of glucocorticoid medications, such as prednisone, is associated with bone loss. These medications affect bone remodeling, leading to increased bone resorption and reduced bone formation.

8. Gender and Body Composition:

- Gender: Women, particularly postmenopausal women, are more prone to osteopenia due to hormonal changes associated with menopause. However, men can also develop osteopenia, especially with advancing age and hormonal changes.

- Body Composition: Low body weight or a small body frame can be a risk factor for osteopenia. Individuals with lower body weight may have less bone mass, making them more susceptible to bone loss.

9. Ethnicity:

Certain ethnic groups may have a higher or lower risk of developing osteopenia. Genetic and environmental factors, including diet and lifestyle, can contribute to variations in bone density among different ethnic populations.

10. History of Fractures:

A history of fractures, especially fragility fractures, may indicate compromised bone health. Individuals who have experienced fractures may be at an increased risk of developing osteopenia or osteoporosis.

Understanding these causes and risk factors is crucial for healthcare providers to assess an individual's risk of developing osteopenia. It allows for targeted interventions, including lifestyle modifications, nutritional interventions, and, in some cases, medication management, to prevent further bone loss and reduce the risk of fractures associated with compromised bone density. Additionally, early identification of osteopenia provides an opportunity for proactive measures to optimize bone health and prevent progression to osteoporosis.

Diagnosis and Assessment:

Diagnosing and assessing osteopenia involves a combination of clinical evaluation, imaging studies, and laboratory tests. The goal is to identify individuals with lower than normal bone mineral density (BMD) and assess their risk of developing osteoporosis and fractures. Here is an overview of the key components of the diagnosis and assessment of osteopenia:

1. Clinical Evaluation:

Clinical evaluation is an essential first step in assessing bone health. Healthcare providers gather information about an individual's medical history, lifestyle, risk factors, and potential symptoms related to bone health. Key components of the clinical evaluation include:

- Medical History: Inquiring about personal and family medical history, including a history of fractures, chronic diseases, hormonal disorders, and medication use.

- Lifestyle Factors: Assessing lifestyle factors such as physical activity, dietary habits (especially calcium and vitamin D intake), smoking history, and alcohol consumption.

- Risk Factors: Identifying specific risk factors for osteopenia, including hormonal changes (such as menopause), age, genetics, and medical conditions that affect bone health.

2. Bone Mineral Density (BMD) Testing:

The gold standard for diagnosing osteopenia is the measurement of bone mineral density through dual-energy X-ray absorptiometry (DXA) scans. DXA is a non-invasive imaging technique that provides precise measurements of BMD at specific sites, commonly the hip and spine. Results are expressed as T-scores, which compare an individual's BMD to that of a healthy young adult.

- T-Score Interpretation:

  - Normal: T-score above -1.0

  - Osteopenia: T-score between -1.0 and -2.5

  - Osteoporosis: T-score -2.5 or lower

The World Health Organization (WHO) defines osteopenia based on T-scores, indicating lower than normal bone density but not to the extent seen in osteoporosis.

3. Quantitative Ultrasound (QUS):

Quantitative ultrasound (QUS) is an alternative method for assessing bone density, particularly at peripheral sites such as the heel. QUS measures the speed of sound through bone and provides an estimation of bone density. While not as precise as DXA, QUS can offer additional insights into bone quality and may be used in certain situations.

4. Laboratory Tests:

Laboratory tests may be conducted to assess specific markers related to bone health and identify potential underlying causes of osteopenia:

- Calcium and Vitamin D Levels: Measurement of serum calcium and vitamin D levels helps identify nutritional deficiencies that can impact bone health.

- Bone Turnover Markers: Blood tests may assess markers of bone turnover, including bone-specific alkaline phosphatase (BALP) and C-terminal telopeptide (CTX). Elevated levels may indicate increased bone turnover associated with osteopenia.

5. Fracture Risk Assessment:

In addition to BMD testing, tools and algorithms are available to assess an individual's risk of fractures. The Fracture Risk Assessment Tool (FRAX) is widely used and incorporates clinical risk factors along with BMD measurements. FRAX provides an estimate of the 10-year probability of major osteoporotic fractures and hip fractures.

6. Imaging Studies:

In certain cases, additional imaging studies may be performed to assess bone health and identify potential causes of bone loss:

- Vertebral Fracture Assessment (VFA): VFA is a specialized imaging technique that assesses the spine for vertebral fractures. It can be performed during a DXA scan and provides valuable information about the presence of fractures.

- Other Imaging Modalities: Complementary imaging studies, such as computed tomography (CT) or magnetic resonance imaging (MRI), may be used to assess bone structure and identify abnormalities.

7. Clinical Risk Factors:

Clinical risk factors for osteopenia include age, gender, family history, hormonal changes (such as menopause), previous fractures, and lifestyle factors. Healthcare providers consider these factors in conjunction with BMD results and fracture risk assessments to formulate a comprehensive understanding of an individual's bone health.

8. Follow-Up and Monitoring:

For individuals diagnosed with osteopenia, regular follow-up and monitoring are essential. Follow-up DXA scans allow healthcare providers to track changes in BMD and assess the effectiveness of preventive interventions. Monitoring may also include assessing for potential side effects of medications, addressing emerging risk factors, and reinforcing lifestyle modifications.

In summary, the diagnosis and assessment of osteopenia involve a combination of clinical evaluation, BMD testing (typically through DXA), laboratory tests, fracture risk assessments, and, in some cases, additional imaging studies. This comprehensive approach allows healthcare providers to identify individuals at risk, assess the severity of bone loss, and implement targeted interventions to prevent further bone loss and reduce the risk of fractures associated with compromised bone density. Early detection and proactive management of osteopenia are crucial for optimizing bone health and preventing progression to osteoporosis.

Clinical Manifestations:

Osteopenia itself does not typically present with specific clinical manifestations or symptoms. Unlike osteoporosis, which can lead to fractures and associated symptoms, osteopenia is often asymptomatic and may go unnoticed by the affected individual. The condition is characterized by lower than normal bone mineral density (BMD) but not to the extent seen in osteoporosis.

While osteopenia may not cause noticeable symptoms, its clinical significance lies in its role as a precursor to osteoporosis. Osteoporosis is a more severe condition characterized by significant bone loss, increased fragility, and an elevated risk of fractures. As osteopenia progresses to

osteoporosis, the risk of fractures, especially hip, spine, and wrist fractures, becomes more pronounced.

Here are some considerations regarding the clinical manifestations of osteopenia:

1. Asymptomatic Nature:

   - Osteopenia is often asymptomatic, meaning individuals with the condition may not experience pain, discomfort, or functional limitations directly related to their bone density.

   - The absence of symptoms makes it challenging for individuals to recognize osteopenia without specific diagnostic testing, such as dual-energy X-ray absorptiometry (DXA) scans.

2. Role as a Precursor to Osteoporosis:

   - Osteopenia serves as an intermediate stage between normal bone density and osteoporosis. It indicates lower-than-optimal bone density but not to the extent that significantly increases the risk of fractures.

   - The clinical significance of osteopenia lies in its potential to progress to osteoporosis, which is associated with a higher risk of fractures and related complications.

3. Increased Fracture Risk:

   - While osteopenia itself may not cause fractures, individuals with osteopenia are at an increased risk of developing fractures compared to those with normal bone density.

   - Fracture risk is particularly elevated if osteopenia progresses to osteoporosis. Common sites for fractures include the hip, spine, and wrist.

4. Bone Health Awareness:

- Individuals diagnosed with osteopenia may become more aware of their bone health and take preventive measures to avoid further bone loss.

- Healthcare providers often use the diagnosis of osteopenia as an opportunity to educate individuals about lifestyle modifications, nutritional interventions, and other strategies to optimize bone health and reduce the risk of fractures.

5. Importance of Monitoring and Intervention:

- Osteopenia highlights the need for monitoring bone health and implementing interventions to prevent further bone loss. Regular follow-up, including repeat dual-energy X-ray absorptiometry (DXA) scans, allows healthcare providers to assess changes in bone density and the effectiveness of preventive measures.

6. Bone Density Testing Recommendations:

- Clinical guidelines often recommend bone density testing, such as DXA scans, for specific populations, including postmenopausal women, men aged 50 and older, and individuals with risk factors for osteoporosis or fractures.

- Identifying osteopenia through these tests helps healthcare providers tailor interventions to manage bone health effectively.

In summary, the clinical manifestations of osteopenia are subtle and often not directly experienced by individuals. Instead, the significance of osteopenia lies in its role as an indicator of compromised bone health, prompting awareness, monitoring, and preventive measures to reduce the risk of fractures and progression to osteoporosis. Early detection and proactive management are essential in optimizing bone health and preventing the potential complications associated with more severe bone loss.

Prevention and Lifestyle Modifications:

Preventing the progression of osteopenia to osteoporosis involves comprehensive lifestyle modifications aimed at optimizing bone health. These interventions are crucial for individuals diagnosed with osteopenia and those at risk of developing compromised bone density.

a. Nutrition and Supplements:

Adequate nutrition, particularly calcium and vitamin D, is essential for maintaining optimal bone health. Calcium is a fundamental component of bone mineralization, and vitamin D facilitates calcium absorption. Dietary sources of calcium include dairy products, leafy green vegetables, and fortified foods. Vitamin D is synthesized through exposure to sunlight, and supplementation may be recommended for individuals with insufficient sun exposure.

b. Weight-Bearing Exercises:

Regular physical activity, especially weight-bearing exercises, is instrumental in preserving and enhancing bone density. Weight-bearing exercises, such as walking, jogging, dancing, and resistance training, stimulate bone formation and help maintain bone mass. Incorporating a variety of exercises that target different muscle groups is beneficial for overall bone health.

c. Smoking Cessation and Limiting Alcohol Intake:

Smoking has detrimental effects on bone health, and quitting smoking is a crucial step in preventing further bone loss. Smoking cessation contributes to improved bone density and reduces the risk of fractures. Similarly, limiting alcohol intake is advisable, as excessive alcohol consumption can interfere with calcium absorption and negatively impact bone health.

d. Fall Prevention Strategies:

Preventing falls is essential for individuals with osteopenia, especially considering the increased risk of fractures associated with compromised bone density. Fall prevention strategies include home safety assessments, addressing environmental hazards, and implementing exercises to improve balance and coordination. Regular eye check-ups and interventions to manage conditions affecting balance are also important components of fall prevention.

e. Medication Management:

In some cases, healthcare providers may recommend medications to prevent further bone loss and reduce the risk of fractures in individuals with osteopenia. Bisphosphonates, selective estrogen receptor modulators (SERMs), and other medications may be prescribed based on individual risk factors and preferences. The decision to initiate medication therapy is made through a thorough assessment of the benefits and potential risks.

Public Health Implications:

Osteopenia, as an intermediate stage between normal bone density and osteoporosis, holds public health implications that extend beyond individual health concerns. Recognizing and addressing osteopenia at a population level can contribute to the overall well-being of communities and reduce the burden associated with osteoporosis-related complications. Here are some key public health implications of osteopenia:

1. Increased Fracture Risk and Healthcare Costs:

   - Osteopenia is associated with an increased risk of fractures, particularly if it progresses to osteoporosis. Fractures, especially hip and vertebral fractures, are associated with significant healthcare costs, including hospitalization, surgery, rehabilitation, and long-term care.

- Public health initiatives targeting osteopenia can potentially reduce the overall economic burden associated with fractures and osteoporosis-related healthcare expenditures.

2. Focus on Prevention and Early Intervention:

- Public health efforts can emphasize prevention and early intervention to address osteopenia proactively. Promoting bone-healthy lifestyles, including adequate nutrition, physical activity, and lifestyle modifications, can contribute to reducing the incidence of osteopenia and its progression to osteoporosis.

- Education campaigns can raise awareness about the importance of bone health and encourage individuals to undergo bone density testing, especially those at higher risk.

3. Implementation of Screening Programs:

- Public health initiatives can advocate for the implementation of bone density screening programs for specific populations, such as postmenopausal women, men aged 50 and older, and individuals with risk factors for osteoporosis.

- Screening programs can help identify osteopenia early, allowing for targeted interventions to prevent further bone loss and reduce the risk of fractures.

4. Promotion of Bone-Healthy Lifestyles:

- Public health campaigns can promote bone-healthy lifestyles, including regular physical activity, a balanced diet rich in calcium and vitamin D, and avoidance of risk factors such as smoking and excessive alcohol consumption.

- Educational programs can target various age groups, emphasizing the importance of building and maintaining optimal bone density throughout the lifespan.

5. Fall Prevention Strategies:

- Osteoporosis and fractures often result from falls, especially in older adults. Public health interventions can focus on fall prevention strategies to reduce the incidence of falls and subsequent fractures.

- Community-based programs, home safety assessments, and educational initiatives can contribute to creating safer environments and reducing fall-related injuries.

6. Ongoing Research and Surveillance:

- Public health agencies can support ongoing research to enhance our understanding of osteopenia, including its prevalence, risk factors, and outcomes. Surveillance systems can help monitor trends in bone health and inform public health strategies.

- Research can also explore the effectiveness of interventions, medications, and lifestyle modifications in preventing the progression of osteopenia and reducing fracture risk.

7. Integration with Chronic Disease Management:

- Osteopenia is often associated with other chronic conditions, such as cardiovascular disease and diabetes. Public health strategies can integrate bone health into broader chronic disease management programs to address the interconnectedness of health conditions.

- Collaborative efforts between healthcare providers, public health agencies, and community organizations can enhance the effectiveness of interventions.

8. Empowerment of At-Risk Populations:

- Public health initiatives can empower at-risk populations, including older adults and individuals with risk factors, to take an active role in managing their bone health.

- Providing accessible information, resources, and support services can empower individuals to make informed decisions about their lifestyles and seek appropriate healthcare interventions.

Addressing osteopenia from a public health perspective involves a comprehensive approach that focuses on prevention, early detection, and the promotion of bone-healthy lifestyles. By integrating bone health into broader public health initiatives and collaborating across healthcare sectors, communities can work towards reducing the impact of osteopenia and osteoporosis on individual health and overall healthcare systems.

Osteopenia represents a critical stage in the continuum of bone health, signaling lower than normal bone mineral density without reaching the threshold for osteoporosis. Understanding the causes, risk factors, diagnosis, and management of osteopenia is essential for healthcare providers, individuals at risk, and the broader community. Preventive strategies, including lifestyle modifications, nutritional interventions, and, in some cases, medication management, play a pivotal role in optimizing bone health and reducing the risk of fractures. Ongoing research and public health initiatives contribute to advancing our understanding of osteopenia and refining approaches to bone health management. Through comprehensive and individualized care, it is possible to address osteopenia proactively, promoting lifelong bone health and reducing the impact of osteoporosis-related complications.

CHAPTER TWO
The Importance of Evidence-Based Approaches

Bone health is a critical aspect of overall well-being, influencing the structural integrity of the skeletal system and playing a vital role in maintaining mobility, independence, and quality of life. As individuals age, the risk of bone-related conditions such as osteoporosis and osteopenia increases, underscoring the importance of effective strategies to optimize bone health. In the field of bone health, evidence-based approaches serve as the cornerstone for guiding interventions, preventive measures, and treatment modalities. This comprehensive exploration delves into the significance of evidence-based approaches in bone health, emphasizing their role in shaping clinical practices, public health initiatives, and individualized patient care.

Evidence-based approaches in healthcare involve integrating the best available scientific evidence with clinical expertise and patient values to inform decision-making. In the context of bone health, evidence-based approaches rely on rigorous scientific research, clinical trials, and systematic reviews to establish a foundation of knowledge. The application of evidence-based principles ensures that interventions and recommendations are grounded in sound scientific reasoning, promoting the most effective and safe practices in the field.

Scientific Rigor and Research Methodology:

Evidence-based approaches in bone health require adherence to rigorous scientific standards and research methodologies. Well-designed clinical trials, systematic reviews, and meta-analyses provide the foundation for generating reliable evidence.

The scientific rigor ensures that interventions are thoroughly evaluated, allowing for the identification of effective strategies, potential risks, and areas requiring further investigation.

Guiding Clinical Practices:

Evidence-based guidelines play a pivotal role in shaping clinical practices related to bone health. These guidelines, often developed by expert panels and organizations, synthesize the available evidence to provide healthcare professionals with recommendations for prevention, diagnosis, and treatment.

Healthcare providers rely on evidence-based guidelines to make informed decisions, tailor interventions to individual patient needs, and optimize outcomes in bone health.

Personalized Medicine in Bone Health:

Evidence-based approaches facilitate personalized medicine in the realm of bone health. Recognizing the heterogeneity among individuals in terms of risk factors, genetics, and responses to interventions, evidence-based practices allow for tailored strategies based on the best available evidence and patient characteristics.

Personalized medicine acknowledges the unique aspects of each patient, ensuring that interventions align with their specific needs, preferences, and health conditions.

Preventive Strategies and Health Promotion:

Evidence-based approaches are instrumental in developing preventive strategies and health promotion initiatives for bone health. Understanding risk factors, lifestyle influences, and the impact of nutrition and physical activity allows for the creation of evidence-based public health campaigns.

Health promotion efforts informed by robust evidence aim to raise awareness, encourage healthy behaviors, and reduce the overall burden of bone-related conditions in populations.

Early Detection and Intervention:

Evidence-based practices emphasize the importance of early detection and intervention in bone health. Screening programs, based on validated diagnostic tools and risk assessment algorithms, enable the identification of individuals at risk of conditions like osteoporosis and osteopenia.

Early intervention, guided by evidence-based guidelines, can prevent or mitigate further bone loss, reducing the likelihood of fractures and associated complications.

Optimizing Treatment Strategies:

Evidence-based approaches guide the selection and optimization of treatment strategies for individuals with compromised bone health. Medications, lifestyle modifications, and therapeutic interventions are evaluated based on their efficacy, safety profile, and impact on patient outcomes.

Clinical decision-making in the treatment of bone-related conditions is enriched by evidence-based practices, ensuring that interventions align with the best available knowledge and contribute to improved patient well-being.

Integration of Nutrition and Lifestyle:

Nutrition and lifestyle factors are integral components of bone health. Evidence-based approaches highlight the relationship between dietary choices, physical activity, and bone density. Nutritional interventions, such as adequate calcium and vitamin D intake, are informed by scientific evidence to support optimal bone health.

Lifestyle recommendations, including weight-bearing exercises, smoking cessation, and moderation of alcohol consumption, are grounded in evidence-based practices to promote skeletal well-being.

Patient Education and Empowerment:

Evidence-based patient education is a key component of promoting bone health. Informing individuals about risk factors, preventive measures, and available interventions empowers them to actively participate in their bone health management.

Patient empowerment through evidence-based education fosters informed decision-making, adherence to recommended strategies, and a sense of autonomy in managing one's bone health.

Advancing Scientific Knowledge:

Evidence-based approaches contribute to the advancement of scientific knowledge in bone health. Ongoing research, supported by evidence-based methodologies, expands our understanding of bone physiology, the impact of genetic factors, and the effectiveness of emerging interventions.

Scientific advancements driven by evidence-based practices lay the groundwork for future innovations, improving the precision and efficacy of interventions in bone health.

Quality Improvement in Healthcare:

Evidence-based practices are integral to quality improvement initiatives in healthcare settings. Healthcare organizations use evidence-based guidelines and protocols to standardize care, enhance patient outcomes, and promote consistency in bone health management.

Quality improvement measures informed by evidence contribute to the delivery of high-quality, patient-centered care across diverse healthcare settings.

Conclusion:

The importance of evidence-based approaches in bone health cannot be overstated. In a field where the consequences of compromised bone health are significant, evidence-based practices provide a robust framework for clinical decision-making, public health initiatives, and individualized patient care. As our understanding of bone physiology and the factors influencing bone health continues to evolve, the reliance on evidence-based approaches becomes increasingly crucial. By integrating the best available scientific evidence with clinical expertise and patient values, the healthcare community can effectively address the challenges posed by conditions such as osteoporosis and osteopenia, ultimately improving the skeletal health and overall well-being of individuals and communities.

CHAPTER THREE

Lifestyle Modifications for Bone Health

Bone health is a vital aspect of overall well-being, influencing an individual's ability to move, support the body's structure, and maintain a high quality of life. While genetics play a role in determining bone density and strength, lifestyle factors also significantly impact bone health. Adopting evidence-based lifestyle modifications is crucial for optimizing bone health, preventing conditions like osteoporosis and osteopenia, and reducing the risk of fractures. This comprehensive exploration delves into the multifaceted realm of lifestyle modifications that contribute to the enhancement of bone health.

Nutritional Considerations:

Nutrition plays a fundamental role in bone health, providing the essential building blocks for bone formation and maintenance. Key nutritional considerations include:

- Calcium Intake: Adequate calcium intake is essential for optimal bone health. Calcium is a primary component of bone, contributing to its strength and density. Dairy products, leafy green vegetables, and fortified foods are excellent sources of calcium.

- Vitamin D: Vitamin D is crucial for calcium absorption and bone mineralization. Exposure to sunlight is a natural source of vitamin D, and dietary sources include fatty fish, fortified dairy products, and supplements as needed.

- Protein: Protein is a vital component of bone tissue. Including sources of lean protein, such as poultry, fish, beans, and nuts, supports bone health and overall musculoskeletal function.

- Phosphorus: Phosphorus, found in foods like meat, dairy, and whole grains, works in conjunction with calcium to maintain bone structure.

- Magnesium: Magnesium is involved in bone metabolism and contributes to bone density. Nuts, seeds, whole grains, and green leafy vegetables are good sources of magnesium.

Weight-Bearing Exercises:

Regular physical activity, particularly weight-bearing exercises, is instrumental in promoting bone health. Weight-bearing exercises stimulate bone remodeling, enhance bone density, and contribute to overall musculoskeletal strength. Examples of weight-bearing exercises include:

- Walking: A simple and effective weight-bearing exercise that can be easily incorporated into daily routines.

- Running and Jogging: Higher-impact activities that promote bone density, especially in the hip and spine.

- Dancing: Engaging in dance routines offers a combination of weight-bearing and aerobic exercise.

- Strength Training: Resistance exercises using weights or resistance bands enhance muscle strength and contribute to bone health.

Smoking Cessation:

Smoking cessation is a crucial component of maintaining optimal bone health. The detrimental effects of smoking on various aspects of health are well-documented, and the skeletal system is no exception. Cigarette smoking has been linked to a range of negative effects on bone density, bone remodeling, and fracture risk. Understanding the relationship between smoking and bone health underscores the importance of smoking cessation as a proactive measure to protect and enhance skeletal well-being.

Smoking has been associated with lower bone density, particularly in the hip and spine. Reduced bone density is a significant risk factor for fractures, as bones become more susceptible to fractures with decreased mineralization. Postmenopausal women who smoke are at a heightened risk of osteoporosis due to hormonal changes and the additional impact of smoking on bone health.

Bone remodeling is a continuous process involving the removal of old bone tissue (resorption) and the formation of new bone tissue. Smoking disrupts this delicate balance, leading to increased bone resorption and decreased bone formation. The net result is a negative impact on bone mass and density, contributing to the development of conditions like osteopenia and osteoporosis.

Smoking has hormonal effects that further compound its impact on bone health. For example, smoking has been linked to lower estrogen levels in women, a hormone crucial for maintaining bone density. Reduced estrogen levels can accelerate bone loss, particularly during menopause, and increase the risk of fractures.

Smoking has been associated with delayed fracture healing. Individuals who smoke may experience prolonged healing times for fractures, increasing the risk of complications and potentially affecting long-term bone health.

Smoking is recognized as a significant independent risk factor for osteoporotic fractures. Osteoporotic fractures, especially hip fractures, are associated with increased morbidity, mortality, and healthcare costs. Smoking cessation is therefore a critical intervention to mitigate this elevated risk.

Smoking can impact blood supply to bones. Adequate blood flow is essential for delivering oxygen and nutrients to bone tissue. Reduced blood supply can compromise bone health and contribute to conditions like avascular necrosis, where bone tissue dies due to a lack of blood supply.

Smoking may interfere with calcium absorption, a crucial process for maintaining bone mineralization. Adequate calcium is necessary for bone strength, and disruptions in absorption can contribute to weakened bones.

Smoking often coexists with other risk factors for bone loss, such as low body weight, inadequate physical activity, and poor nutritional habits. The synergistic impact of smoking with these factors can exacerbate the risk of bone-related conditions.

Smoking not only affects bone density but also influences bone quality and microarchitecture. Changes in bone microarchitecture, including alterations in trabecular bone structure, contribute to increased fragility and fracture risk.

Secondhand smoke exposure, particularly in childhood and adolescence, can have lasting effects on bone health. Individuals exposed to secondhand smoke may experience compromised bone density and an increased risk of fractures later in life.

One encouraging aspect is that many of the negative effects of smoking on bone health are reversible with smoking cessation. Quitting smoking can lead to improvements in bone density, albeit over time, and contribute to a reduction in fracture risk.

Successful smoking cessation is often part of a multifaceted approach to bone health. Combining efforts to quit smoking with strategies such as weight-bearing exercises, adequate nutrition, and other lifestyle modifications enhances the overall impact on bone health.

In conclusion, smoking cessation is a critical and achievable step toward maintaining and improving bone health. The detrimental effects of smoking on bone density, remodeling, hormonal balance, and fracture risk underscore the importance of quitting smoking as a proactive measure. Individuals seeking to optimize their bone health should consider smoking cessation as an integral part of a comprehensive strategy that includes lifestyle modifications, nutritional interventions, and regular health check-ups. The benefits of quitting smoking extend far beyond respiratory health, positively impacting the entire musculoskeletal system and contributing to a higher quality of life.

Limiting Alcohol Consumption:

Limiting alcohol consumption is an important lifestyle modification that positively influences bone health. While moderate alcohol intake may not have significant adverse effects, excessive and chronic alcohol consumption has been associated with an increased risk of bone-related conditions, including osteoporosis and fractures. Understanding the impact of alcohol on bone health and the benefits of limiting consumption is crucial for individuals seeking to maintain strong and healthy bones.

Excessive alcohol intake can interfere with the body's ability to absorb calcium, a critical mineral for bone health. Calcium is an essential component of bone tissue, contributing to its strength and density. Impaired calcium absorption can compromise bone mineralization and increase the risk of osteoporosis.

Chronic alcohol consumption has been linked to lower bone density. Reduced bone density is a key factor in the development of osteoporosis, a condition characterized by fragile and porous bones that are more susceptible to fractures.

Alcohol can disrupt hormonal balance, particularly affecting sex hormones such as estrogen and testosterone. Hormonal imbalances contribute to accelerated bone loss, especially in postmenopausal women, and increase the risk of fractures.

Individuals with a history of heavy alcohol consumption are at an increased risk of fractures. Alcohol-related falls and accidents can result in fractures, and compromised bone density exacerbates the severity of these fractures.

Chronic alcohol consumption contributes to a phenomenon known as alcohol-induced bone loss. This condition involves increased bone resorption (the breakdown of bone tissue) and decreased bone formation, leading to a negative impact on overall bone mass.

Excessive alcohol intake has been associated with vitamin D deficiency. Vitamin D is crucial for calcium absorption and bone health. Deficiency in vitamin D can contribute to weakened bones and an increased risk of fractures.

Alcohol consumption can adversely affect bone microarchitecture, including changes in trabecular bone structure. These alterations in bone microarchitecture contribute to increased fragility and fracture risk.

Osteoblasts are cells responsible for bone formation. Chronic alcohol consumption can inhibit the function of osteoblasts, leading to impaired bone-building processes and compromised bone strength.

Alcohol is a diuretic, leading to increased urine production and potential dehydration. Dehydration can affect electrolyte balance, disrupting the minerals necessary for bone health, including calcium and phosphorus.

The negative effects of alcohol on bone health can be compounded when combined with other risk factors, such as smoking. Smoking and heavy alcohol consumption together may have a synergistic impact, further increasing the risk of bone-related conditions.

The good news is that many of the negative effects of alcohol on bone health are reversible with the limitation or cessation of alcohol consumption. Adopting a lifestyle that includes moderation in alcohol intake can contribute to improvements in bone density and overall skeletal health.

While excessive alcohol consumption poses risks to bone health, moderate alcohol intake may not have the same detrimental effects. Moderation is often defined as up to one drink per day for women and up to two drinks per day for men. This level of consumption is generally considered acceptable and may not have significant negative impacts on bone health.

In conclusion, limiting alcohol consumption is a prudent strategy for maintaining and enhancing bone health. Understanding the complex relationship between alcohol and bone health empowers individuals to make informed decisions about their lifestyle choices. By adopting a balanced approach to alcohol intake, individuals can contribute to the preservation of bone density, reduce the risk of fractures, and promote overall musculoskeletal well-being. It is essential for individuals to consider alcohol consumption as part of a broader commitment to a healthy lifestyle that includes proper nutrition, regular physical activity, and other bone-protective measures.

Balanced Diet and Maintaining a Healthy Body Weight:

Achieving and maintaining a healthy body weight is essential for bone health. Extreme weight loss, especially through restrictive diets, can lead to bone loss and increased fracture risk. A balanced diet that provides essential nutrients supports overall health, including bone health.

Fall Prevention Strategies:

Falls are a significant risk factor for fractures, especially in older adults. Implementing fall prevention strategies is crucial to protect bone health and reduce the likelihood of fractures. Strategies include:

- Home Safety Assessments: Identifying and addressing potential hazards in the home environment to prevent falls.

- Balance Exercises: Engaging in exercises that improve balance and coordination reduces the risk of falls.

- Regular Eye Check-ups: Ensuring optimal vision contributes to a person's ability to navigate their environment safely.

Stress Management:

Chronic stress can negatively impact bone health. Stress hormones, such as cortisol, may contribute to bone loss. Incorporating stress management techniques, such as mindfulness, meditation, and relaxation exercises, into daily routines can promote overall well-being, including bone health.

Adequate Hydration:

Adequate hydration is a crucial factor for maintaining overall health, and it also plays a role in supporting bone health. While the direct impact of hydration on bones may not be as well-known as other factors, such as calcium intake and physical activity, staying well-hydrated is essential for various physiological processes that indirectly influence bone health. Here are several ways in which adequate hydration contributes to bone health:

1. Nutrient Transport: Water is a fundamental component of blood, and blood is responsible for transporting nutrients, including those vital for bone health. Nutrients like calcium, phosphorus, and magnesium, which are essential for bone formation and maintenance, rely on proper hydration for efficient transport to bone tissues.

2. Electrolyte Balance: Electrolytes, including calcium, potassium, and sodium, play a crucial role in bone health. Maintaining proper electrolyte balance is essential for bone metabolism and overall cellular function. Hydration supports the balance of these electrolytes, contributing to optimal bone health.

3. Calcium Metabolism: Adequate hydration is associated with improved calcium metabolism. Water helps dissolve and transport calcium in the body, facilitating its absorption in the intestines and aiding in the formation of hydroxyapatite, a key component of bone tissue.

4. Joint Lubrication: Proper hydration helps maintain joint health by ensuring adequate lubrication of joints. This is particularly relevant for the joints surrounding bones, providing support and reducing the risk of injuries that could impact bone health.

5. Waste Removal: Hydration is essential for the removal of waste products from the body. Efficient waste removal prevents the accumulation of substances that could interfere with bone metabolism and contribute to conditions that affect bone health.

6. Temperature Regulation: Maintaining an appropriate body temperature is crucial for overall health. Water is a primary component of sweat, which plays a key role in cooling the body during physical activity. Engaging in regular physical activity is beneficial for bone health, and adequate hydration supports the body's ability to regulate temperature during exercise.

7. Prevention of Dehydration-Related Complications: Severe dehydration can lead to complications that indirectly impact bone health. For example, kidney stones, which are more

likely to occur in dehydrated individuals, can affect the balance of minerals in the body, including those important for bone health.

8. Enhancing Physical Performance: Staying well-hydrated is essential for maintaining physical performance, including engaging in weight-bearing exercises that promote bone density. Dehydration can lead to fatigue, decreased endurance, and impaired physical function, which may negatively affect bone health over time.

9. Impact on Bone Microarchitecture: While research on this aspect is ongoing, some studies suggest that dehydration may have subtle effects on bone microarchitecture. Maintaining adequate hydration levels could contribute to preserving bone structure.

10. Complementing Other Bone-Healthy Habits: Hydration is one component of an overall healthy lifestyle that supports bone health. When combined with proper nutrition, weight-bearing exercises, and other bone-protective measures, adequate hydration contributes to a comprehensive approach to maintaining strong and resilient bones.

Tips for Adequate Hydration:

- Drink water regularly throughout the day.

- Consider factors such as climate, physical activity level, and individual health needs when determining hydration requirements.

- Be mindful of signs of dehydration, such as dark urine, thirst, and dry mouth.

- Consume water-rich foods, such as fruits and vegetables, as part of your diet.

In summary, while hydration may not be the sole determinant of bone health, it is a critical factor that influences various processes in the body, including those related to bone metabolism. Staying well-hydrated complements other bone-healthy habits and contributes to overall well-being. Individuals striving to maintain optimal bone health should prioritize adequate hydration as part of a holistic approach to a healthy lifestyle.

Regular Health Check-ups:

Regular health check-ups are a cornerstone of proactive healthcare, playing a crucial role in safeguarding bone health. These routine examinations and assessments offer a comprehensive view of an individual's musculoskeletal well-being, providing opportunities for early detection, prevention, and intervention. Key components of health check-ups for bone health include:

1. Bone Density Testing:

   - Purpose: To assess bone mineral density and identify potential risks of osteoporosis or fractures.

   - Method: Dual-Energy X-ray Absorptiometry (DEXA) scans are commonly used for precise measurements.

2. Physical Examination:

   - Purpose: To evaluate joint health, flexibility, and detect any signs of musculoskeletal issues.

   - Assessment: Healthcare professionals examine joints, range of motion, and signs of deformities.

3. Blood Tests:

   - Purpose: To assess levels of essential nutrients (calcium, vitamin D) and hormones influencing bone health.

   - Markers: Calcium and vitamin D levels, parathyroid hormone (PTH), and sex hormones.

4. Evaluation of Risk Factors:

   - Purpose: To identify individual factors such as age, family history, and lifestyle that may impact bone health.

   - Outcome: Tailoring preventive measures and interventions based on identified risks.

5. Medication Review:

   - Purpose: To review medications for potential impact on bone health.

   - Focus: Identifying medications, such as steroids, that may contribute to bone loss.

6. Nutritional Assessment:

   - Purpose: To identify nutrient deficiencies or imbalances affecting bone health.

   - Focus: Ensuring adequate intake of calcium, vitamin D, and other essential nutrients.

7. Lifestyle Factors:

- Purpose: To assess lifestyle choices influencing bone health, such as physical activity, smoking, and alcohol consumption.

   - Recommendations: Guidance on adopting bone-protective behaviors.

8. Falls Risk Assessment:

   - Purpose: Particularly for older adults, to assess the risk of falls that may lead to fractures.

   - Outcome: Identifying and addressing factors contributing to falls.

9. Bone Health Education:

   - Purpose: To provide individuals with information on bone health importance and preventive measures.

   - Empowerment: Educating individuals to make informed decisions for bone-protective behaviors.

10. Follow-up and Monitoring:

   - Purpose: To ensure ongoing monitoring of bone health and identify any changes.

   - Action: Timely intervention and adjustments to the healthcare plan.

11. Screening for Other Health Conditions:

   - Purpose: Identifying conditions that may impact bone health, such as rheumatoid arthritis or hormonal disorders.

   - Holistic Approach: Ensuring comprehensive care by addressing underlying health factors.

12. Personalized Plans:

   - Outcome: Developing personalized plans based on health check-up results.

   - Components: Recommendations for nutrition, exercise, and lifestyle modifications for optimal bone health.

In essence, regular health check-ups for bone health serve as a proactive and personalized approach to maintaining the integrity of the skeletal system. These assessments contribute to early intervention, risk mitigation, and the empowerment of individuals in actively managing their bone health for a resilient and strong musculoskeletal structure.

Hormonal Health:

Hormonal imbalances, particularly in relation to estrogen and testosterone, can affect bone health. Addressing hormonal health through appropriate medical interventions, lifestyle changes, and, when necessary, hormone replacement therapy, contributes to maintaining bone density.

Limiting High-Caffeine Intake:

Limiting high-caffeine intake is a consideration for promoting optimal bone health. While moderate caffeine consumption is generally considered safe and may even have some health benefits, excessive intake could potentially impact bone density. Here's a brief overview of the relationship between high caffeine intake and bone health:

1. Calcium Absorption Interference: High caffeine intake has been associated with increased calcium excretion in the urine. Calcium is a vital mineral for bone health, and when excessive amounts are lost through urine, it can potentially contribute to reduced calcium availability for bone maintenance.

2. Negative Impact on Bone Density: Some studies suggest a potential negative association between high caffeine consumption and bone density. Excessive caffeine intake may interfere with the process of bone mineralization, potentially leading to lower bone density.

3. Potential Hormonal Effects: Caffeine consumption may influence hormones such as parathyroid hormone (PTH) and cortisol, which play roles in bone metabolism. Changes in these hormonal levels could impact bone health, although the exact mechanisms are still being studied.

4. Risk of Osteoporotic Fractures: Some research indicates that high caffeine intake, particularly in postmenopausal women, may be associated with an increased risk of osteoporotic fractures. This risk may be more pronounced in individuals with low calcium intake.

5. Moderation as a Key Strategy: While the evidence is not conclusive, moderation in caffeine intake is often recommended. Moderation can help strike a balance between enjoying the potential benefits of caffeine, such as improved alertness, and minimizing any potential negative effects on bone health.

6. Dietary Sources of Caffeine: Caffeine is commonly found in coffee, tea, energy drinks, and certain sodas. Being mindful of total daily caffeine intake, including both beverages and foods, is important for those concerned about bone health.

7. Individual Sensitivity: Individual responses to caffeine can vary. Some people may be more sensitive to the potential bone-related effects of caffeine. It's essential to consider personal factors and consult with healthcare professionals for personalized advice.

8. Importance of Calcium-Rich Foods: To counterbalance the potential impact of caffeine on calcium absorption, it's crucial to ensure an adequate intake of calcium-rich foods. Dairy products, leafy green vegetables, and fortified foods can contribute to maintaining sufficient calcium levels.

9. Consideration for Specific Populations: Certain populations, such as postmenopausal women and older adults, may be more vulnerable to the potential bone-related effects of excessive caffeine intake. Consulting with healthcare providers can help tailor recommendations based on individual needs.

While research on the relationship between high caffeine intake and bone health is ongoing, there is some evidence to suggest a potential association. Adopting a balanced approach by moderating caffeine intake and ensuring adequate calcium intake through a well-balanced diet is a prudent strategy. As with many aspects of health, individual factors play a role, and personalized advice from healthcare professionals is valuable for making informed decisions about caffeine consumption and its potential impact on bone health.

Awareness of Medication Effects:

Being aware of the potential effects of medications on bone health is crucial for maintaining overall well-being. Certain medications may impact bone density and increase the risk of bone-related conditions, such as osteoporosis and fractures. Here's a brief overview of the importance of being mindful of medication effects on bone health:

1. Steroids and Bone Loss: Corticosteroids, often prescribed for inflammatory conditions like arthritis, asthma, or autoimmune disorders, are known to contribute to bone loss. Long-term use of these medications may increase the risk of osteoporosis and fractures.

2. Antacids and Proton Pump Inhibitors (PPIs): Some antacids and PPIs, used to manage conditions like acid reflux and heartburn, may interfere with calcium absorption. Calcium is crucial for bone health, and reduced absorption can impact bone density.

3. Antidepressants and Antipsychotics: Certain antidepressants and antipsychotic medications may have side effects that affect bone metabolism. It's essential to discuss potential bone health implications with healthcare providers when considering or using these medications.

4. Hormonal Therapies: Hormonal therapies, including some treatments for breast and prostate cancers, may have effects on bone density. Estrogen and testosterone play roles in maintaining bone health, and alterations in hormone levels can impact bone metabolism.

5. Thyroid Medications: Thyroid medications, when not properly regulated, can influence bone health. Both hypothyroidism and hyperthyroidism can have implications for bone density.

6. Awareness of Medication Interactions: Some medications may interact with each other, potentially affecting bone health. It's essential to inform healthcare providers about all medications, including over-the-counter drugs and supplements, to assess potential interactions.

7. Ongoing Monitoring and Adjustments: Regular check-ups with healthcare providers allow for ongoing monitoring of medication effects on bone health. Adjustments to medication regimens or additional interventions may be considered to mitigate any adverse effects.

8. Individualized Approaches: Medication effects on bone health can vary from person to person. Healthcare providers consider individual health profiles, including age, gender, and existing medical conditions, to tailor treatment plans that minimize potential risks to bone health.

9. Communication with Healthcare Providers: Open and transparent communication with healthcare providers is essential. Patients should discuss any concerns about medication effects on bone health and inquire about strategies to mitigate potential risks.

10. Lifestyle Modifications: For individuals on medications that may impact bone health, adopting lifestyle modifications becomes crucial. This may include ensuring an adequate intake of bone-supportive nutrients, engaging in weight-bearing exercises, and avoiding other lifestyle factors that contribute to bone loss.

Awareness of medication effects on bone health is a proactive step toward maintaining skeletal well-being. Individuals taking medications with potential implications for bone health should engage in ongoing discussions with their healthcare providers. This collaborative approach allows for the careful balancing of treatment benefits with potential risks to ensure overall health and the preservation of bone density.

In conclusion, lifestyle modifications play a pivotal role in promoting and maintaining optimal bone health throughout the lifespan. From nutrition and physical activity to smoking cessation, fall prevention, and stress management, these evidence-based strategies contribute to the prevention of conditions like osteoporosis and osteopenia. Recognizing the interconnectedness of lifestyle choices and their impact on bone health empowers individuals to make informed decisions and actively participate in preserving their musculoskeletal well-being. Implementing comprehensive lifestyle modifications not only supports bone health but also contributes to overall health and longevity. Through a holistic approach that addresses both individual behaviors and broader public health initiatives, the promotion of bone health becomes an integral component of a comprehensive healthcare strategy.

CHAPTER FOUR

Nutrition and Its Impact on Bone Density

Nutrition plays a pivotal role in maintaining bone health, influencing bone density, and preventing conditions such as osteoporosis. The human skeleton undergoes constant remodeling, a process that involves the breakdown of old bone tissue and the formation of new bone. Nutrients from the diet provide the building blocks for this dynamic process, ensuring the strength, density, and integrity of bones throughout life. In this comprehensive exploration, we delve into the intricate relationship between nutrition and bone density, examining the key nutrients, dietary patterns, and lifestyle factors that contribute to optimal skeletal health.

Calcium: The Foundation of Bone Health

Calcium stands as the cornerstone of bone health, comprising a significant portion of bone mineral. It plays a vital role in bone formation, providing the structural framework for bones and teeth. The body tightly regulates calcium levels, primarily in collaboration with vitamin D and parathyroid hormone.

Dietary Sources:

- Dairy products: Milk, cheese, yogurt

- Leafy green vegetables: Kale, broccoli, bok choy

- Fortified foods: Certain cereals, juices, and plant-based milk alternatives

Impact on Bone Density:

Adequate calcium intake during childhood and adolescence is crucial for achieving peak bone mass, laying the foundation for lifelong bone health. In adulthood, calcium maintains bone density and helps counteract age-related bone loss. Insufficient calcium intake may lead to weakened bones, increasing the risk of fractures and osteoporosis.

Vitamin D: Calcium's Facilitator

Vitamin D is essential for calcium absorption in the intestines, a process vital for maintaining proper calcium levels in the blood. The skin synthesizes vitamin D upon exposure to sunlight, but dietary sources and supplements also contribute significantly.

Dietary Sources:

- Fatty fish: Salmon, mackerel, tuna

- Fortified foods: Milk, orange juice, cereals

- Egg yolks

Impact on Bone Density:

Vitamin D deficiency can hinder calcium absorption, compromising bone health. In severe cases, it can lead to conditions like rickets in children and osteomalacia in adults. Maintaining sufficient vitamin D levels supports calcium metabolism, contributing to optimal bone density.

Phosphorus and Magnesium: Collaborators in Bone Structure

Phosphorus, like calcium, is a key mineral in bone composition, forming the mineralized matrix that provides bone strength. Magnesium plays a role in bone structure and function, influencing bone mineralization and supporting the activity of enzymes involved in bone metabolism.

Dietary Sources:

- Phosphorus: Meat, dairy products, nuts, and seeds

- Magnesium: Whole grains, nuts, leafy green vegetables, legumes

Impact on Bone Density:

Balancing phosphorus intake with calcium is essential for optimal bone health. Magnesium contributes to bone density by supporting the formation of hydroxyapatite, the mineral complex that provides strength to bones. Imbalances in these minerals may affect bone metabolism.

Protein: The Building Blocks of Bone Tissue

Protein is a fundamental component of bone tissue, providing the amino acids necessary for bone formation and maintenance. Collagen, a major protein in bones, gives them flexibility and resilience.

Dietary Sources:

- Lean meats: Chicken, turkey, fish

- Dairy products: Milk, yogurt, cheese

- Plant-based sources: Beans, lentils, tofu, nuts

Impact on Bone Density:

Adequate protein intake supports bone health by providing the necessary amino acids for collagen synthesis. However, excessively high protein intake, particularly from animal sources, may increase calcium excretion and potentially impact bone density. Striking a balance is crucial for optimizing bone health.

Vitamin K: Regulating Calcium in Bones

Vitamin K plays a vital role in bone metabolism by regulating calcium within bone tissues. It is involved in the synthesis of osteocalcin, a protein that helps bind calcium to the bone matrix.

Dietary Sources:

- Leafy green vegetables: Kale, spinach, broccoli

- Cruciferous vegetables: Brussels sprouts, cabbage

- Fermented foods: Natto, a Japanese dish made from fermented soybeans

Impact on Bone Density:

Adequate vitamin K levels contribute to bone health by supporting the proper incorporation of calcium into bone tissue. Deficiencies in vitamin K may impair bone mineralization and increase the risk of fractures.

Boron: Enhancing Bone Health

While boron's role in bone health is not as well-studied as other minerals, it is believed to play a role in bone development and maintenance. Boron may influence bone metabolism by interacting with hormones and enzymes involved in calcium and magnesium metabolism.

Dietary Sources:

- Nuts: Almonds, walnuts

- Legumes: Beans, lentils

- Fruits: Apples, oranges, grapes

Impact on Bone Density:

Research on boron's impact on bone health is ongoing, but some studies suggest a potential positive association between boron intake and bone density. Including boron-rich foods in the diet may contribute to overall bone health.

Vitamin C: Collagen Synthesis for Bone Strength

Vitamin C is essential for collagen synthesis, a crucial process for maintaining the strength and integrity of bones. Collagen provides the organic matrix in which minerals like calcium and phosphorus are deposited.

Dietary Sources:

- Citrus fruits: Oranges, lemons, grapefruits

- Beries: Strawberries, blueberries, raspberries

- Vegetables: Bell peppers, broccoli, spinach

Impact on Bone Density:

Adequate vitamin C intake supports the formation of collagen, contributing to the tensile strength of bones. It also aids in the absorption of non-heme iron from plant-based foods, further supporting overall bone health.

Zinc: Enzyme Function in Bone Metabolism

Zinc is involved in the activity of enzymes that play a role in bone metabolism. It supports the function of alkaline phosphatase, an enzyme that participates in bone mineralization.

Dietary Sources:

- Meat: Beef, pork, lamb

- Shellfish: Crab, lobster, shrimp

- Legumes: Lentils, chickpeas

Impact on Bone Density:

Zinc deficiency may compromise bone health by affecting the activity of enzymes involved in bone metabolism. Ensuring sufficient zinc intake supports these enzymatic processes, contributing to optimal bone density.

Copper: Collagen Formation and Cross-Linking

Copper is involved in the formation and cross-linking of collagen, the protein that provides flexibility and strength to bones. It plays a role in the synthesis of connective tissues, including those in bones.

Dietary Sources:

- Shellfish: Oysters, crab, lobster

- Nuts and seeds: Cashews, sunflower seeds

- Whole grains: Quinoa, oats

Impact on Bone Density:

Copper contributes to bone health by supporting the formation of collagen fibers. While copper deficiency is rare, maintaining an adequate intake of this trace mineral is essential for overall bone strength.

Iron: Oxygen Transport and Bone Health

Iron is crucial for transporting oxygen in the blood, supporting metabolic processes in bone cells. It is involved in the synthesis of collagen and other proteins necessary for bone structure.

Dietary Sources:

- Red meat: Beef, lamb, pork

- Poultry: Chicken, turkey

- Plant-based sources: Lentils, beans, spinach

Impact on Bone Density:

Iron deficiency anemia may affect bone health by impairing collagen synthesis. However, excessive iron intake may also have negative effects. Striking a balance and ensuring proper iron levels contribute to overall bone health.

Omega-3 Fatty Acids: Balancing Inflammation

Omega-3 fatty acids, especially EPA (eicosapentaenoic acid) and DHA (docosahexaenoic acid), play a role in modulating inflammation. Chronic inflammation can negatively impact bone health, and omega-3s contribute to a balanced inflammatory response.

Dietary Sources:

- Fatty fish: Salmon, mackerel, sardines

- Flaxseeds and chia seeds

- Walnuts

Impact on Bone Density:

While research on omega-3s and bone health is ongoing, their anti-inflammatory properties may indirectly support bone density by mitigating chronic inflammation. Including omega-3-rich foods in the diet promotes overall musculoskeletal well-being.

Anti-Inflammatory Diet: Reducing Bone Stress

Chronic inflammation is associated with conditions that affect bone health, including osteoporosis. Adopting an anti-inflammatory diet rich in fruits, vegetables, whole grains, and omega-3 fatty acids may help mitigate inflammation and support optimal bone density.

Dietary Recommendations:

- Colorful fruits and vegetables: Berries, leafy greens, tomatoes

- Whole grains: Quinoa, brown rice, oats

- Healthy fats: Olive oil, avocados, nuts

Impact on Bone Density:

An anti-inflammatory diet focuses on nutrient-dense, whole foods that provide a range of vitamins and minerals crucial for bone health. By reducing inflammation, this dietary approach supports the preservation of bone density.

Lifestyle Factors: Beyond the Plate

Beyond dietary choices, lifestyle factors significantly contribute to bone health. Incorporating weight-bearing exercises, such as walking, running, and strength training, stimulates bone remodeling, promoting the retention of bone density. Adequate exposure to sunlight ensures the synthesis of vitamin D, a key player in calcium absorption.

Exercise and Bone Density:

- Weight-bearing exercises: Walking, jogging, dancing

- Strength training: Resistance exercises, weightlifting

- Flexibility exercises: Yoga, Pilates

Sunlight Exposure:

- Aim for 10-30 minutes of sunlight exposure several times a week

- Factors like skin type, time of day, and geographic location influence vitamin D synthesis

Bone Health Throughout the Lifespan

Childhood and Adolescence:

- Focus: Achieving peak bone mass

- Nutritional Emphasis: Adequate calcium and vitamin D intake, along with a balanced diet

  - Activities: Encouraging physical activity and weight-bearing exercises

Adulthood:

  - Focus: Maintaining bone density and preventing age-related bone loss

  - Nutritional Emphasis: Balanced diet with sufficient calcium, vitamin D, and other bone-supportive nutrients

  - Activities: Incorporating weight-bearing exercises and staying physically active

Older Adults:

  - Focus: Preventing fractures and preserving bone density

  - Nutritional Emphasis: Adequate protein, calcium, vitamin D, and other nutrients for bone health

  - Activities: Weight-bearing exercises, balance training, and fall prevention strategies

Special Considerations: Bone Health and Women

Women face unique considerations related to bone health, particularly during periods such as pregnancy, lactation, and menopause. During pregnancy and lactation, calcium and vitamin D needs increase to support the developing fetus and ensure optimal bone health for both the mother and the infant. Menopause brings hormonal changes, with a decline in estrogen levels contributing to accelerated bone loss. Addressing these life stages requires tailored nutritional strategies and lifestyle adjustments.

Pregnancy and Lactation:

  - Nutritional Emphasis: Increased calcium and vitamin D intake

  - Activities: Safe and appropriate physical activity during pregnancy, including exercises that support bone health

Menopause:

   - Nutritional Emphasis: Adequate calcium and vitamin D intake, and consideration of supplements

   - Activities: Weight-bearing exercises, strength training, and activities that promote balance and flexibility

Common Myths and Misconceptions

1. Myth: Dairy is the Only Source of Calcium

- While dairy products are rich in calcium, there are various non-dairy sources, such as leafy green vegetables, fortified foods, and certain fish.

2. Myth: Supplements Alone Suffice for Bone Health

- Supplements can be beneficial, but they should complement a balanced diet. Nutrients interact synergistically in food, and relying solely on supplements may miss out on these interactions.

3. Myth: Only Older Adults Need to Worry About Bone Health

- Building and maintaining optimal bone density is a lifelong process. Ensuring adequate nutrition and engaging in bone-supportive activities are important at every stage of life.

4. Myth: Bone Health Is Solely Determined by Genetics

- While genetics play a role, lifestyle factors, including nutrition and physical activity, significantly influence bone health. Healthy habits can mitigate genetic predispositions.

Challenges and Solutions: Overcoming Barriers to Optimal Bone Health

Achieving and maintaining optimal bone health involves overcoming various challenges, from dietary considerations to lifestyle factors. Understanding and addressing these challenges is essential for preventing conditions like osteoporosis and fractures. Here, we explore common obstacles to optimal bone health and propose solutions to overcome them.

1. Insufficient Calcium Intake:

   - Challenge: Many individuals do not meet the recommended daily intake of calcium, a crucial mineral for bone health.

   - Solution: Encouraging the consumption of calcium-rich foods such as dairy products, leafy green vegetables, fortified plant-based milk, and fish with edible bones. Additionally, calcium supplements may be considered under the guidance of healthcare providers.

2. Vitamin D Deficiency:

   - Challenge: Inadequate exposure to sunlight and insufficient dietary intake contribute to vitamin D deficiencies.

   - Solution: Promoting moderate sun exposure, especially in regions with limited sunlight, and incorporating vitamin D-rich foods (e.g., fatty fish, fortified products) into the diet. Vitamin D supplements may be recommended, particularly for individuals with limited sun exposure or specific health conditions.

3. Poor Dietary Habits:

   - Challenge: Unhealthy dietary habits, such as excessive consumption of processed foods, sugary beverages, and inadequate intake of nutrient-dense foods, can negatively impact bone health.

   - Solution: Promoting balanced and diverse diets that include a variety of fruits, vegetables, whole grains, lean proteins, and dairy or dairy alternatives. Nutrition education and awareness campaigns can play a pivotal role in encouraging healthier eating habits.

4. Sedentary Lifestyle:

   - Challenge: Lack of physical activity, particularly weight-bearing exercises, contributes to decreased bone density.

   - Solution: Encouraging regular physical activity that includes weight-bearing exercises, such as walking, running, and strength training. Promoting physical education in schools and creating

community programs that emphasize bone-strengthening activities can help address this
challenge.

5. Smoking and Excessive Alcohol Consumption:

   - Challenge: Smoking and excessive alcohol intake are known risk factors for bone loss and
fractures.

   - Solution: Implementing public health campaigns to raise awareness of the detrimental effects
of smoking and excessive alcohol consumption on bone health. Providing support programs for
smoking cessation and alcohol moderation can contribute to improved bone health.

6. Aging Population:

   - Challenge: Aging is associated with natural declines in bone density, making older adults
more susceptible to fractures.

   - Solution: Implementing preventive measures early in life, such as promoting bone-healthy
habits in childhood and adolescence. For older adults, encouraging regular physical activity, a
nutrient-rich diet, and addressing specific age-related challenges through tailored healthcare
strategies.

7. Dietary Restrictions:

   - Challenge: Individuals with dietary restrictions, such as lactose intolerance or vegetarianism,
may face challenges in obtaining sufficient bone-supportive nutrients.

   - Solution: Providing personalized dietary guidance to address nutrient gaps based on
individual dietary preferences and restrictions. Encouraging the inclusion of alternative calcium
and vitamin D sources, such as fortified plant-based products.

8. Digestive Disorders:

   - Challenge: Conditions affecting nutrient absorption, such as celiac disease or inflammatory
bowel diseases, can impact bone health.

   - Solution: Managing digestive disorders through appropriate medical care and dietary
adjustments. Collaboration between healthcare providers and nutritionists can help individuals
with these conditions maintain optimal bone health.

9. Socioeconomic Disparities:

   - Challenge: Socioeconomic factors can influence access to nutritious foods, healthcare resources, and opportunities for physical activity.

   - Solution: Implementing community-based initiatives to address socioeconomic disparities, such as providing access to affordable, nutrient-dense foods, and creating programs that make physical activity accessible to diverse populations.

10. Lack of Awareness:

   - Challenge: Many individuals may lack awareness of the importance of bone health and preventive measures.

   - Solution: Launching public health campaigns to educate the general population about the significance of bone health, emphasizing the role of nutrition, physical activity, and lifestyle choices. Integrating bone health education into school curricula can help instill lifelong habits.

11. Nutrient Interactions and Individual Variability:

   - Challenge: Nutrient interactions and individual variability in nutrient needs pose challenges to providing one-size-fits-all recommendations.

   - Solution: Emphasizing the importance of a well-balanced diet that includes a variety of nutrient-rich foods. Encouraging individuals to consult with healthcare providers or registered dietitians for personalized advice based on their unique health profiles and needs.

12. Accessibility to Healthcare:

   - Challenge: Limited access to healthcare resources may hinder individuals from receiving timely preventive care and nutritional guidance.

   - Solution: Advocating for improved access to healthcare services, especially preventive care focused on bone health. Implementing telehealth options and community-based healthcare initiatives can enhance accessibility.

13. Incorporating Bone Health into Primary Care:

   - Challenge: Bone health may not always be prioritized in primary care settings.

   - Solution: Promoting the integration of bone health assessments and preventive measures into routine primary care. Healthcare providers can routinely inquire about dietary habits, physical activity, and other lifestyle factors that impact bone health during patient visits.

14. Multidisciplinary Approach:

   - Challenge: Optimal bone health requires a multidisciplinary approach that involves healthcare providers, nutritionists, educators, and community leaders.

   - Solution: Fostering collaboration between various stakeholders to develop comprehensive strategies for promoting bone health. Integrating bone health education into healthcare systems, schools, and community programs can create a holistic and synergistic approach.

15. Research and Policy Advocacy:

   - Challenge: Limited research on certain aspects of bone health and inadequate policy support for preventive measures.

   - Solution: Advocating for increased research funding to further understand the complexities of bone health. Engaging policymakers to develop and support initiatives that prioritize bone health education, preventive measures, and access to resources.

In conclusion, overcoming challenges to optimal bone health requires a multifaceted and collaborative approach. From promoting healthier lifestyles to addressing socioeconomic disparities and raising awareness, concerted efforts at individual, community, and societal levels are essential. By implementing evidence-based strategies, integrating bone health into routine healthcare practices, and fostering public awareness, we can work towards a future where individuals of all ages maintain strong and resilient bones, reducing the burden of bone-related conditions and improving overall well-being.

CHAPTER FIVE

Weight-Bearing Exercises for Stronger Bones

Maintaining strong and healthy bones is crucial for overall well-being, and weight-bearing exercises play a pivotal role in achieving and sustaining optimal bone health. Bones are dynamic tissues that respond to mechanical stress by becoming denser and stronger. Weight-bearing exercises, also known as resistance or strength training, involve working against gravity to create stress on the bones, ultimately promoting bone growth and density. In this comprehensive exploration, we delve into the significance of weight-bearing exercises for bone health, the mechanisms behind their effectiveness, and the diverse range of exercises that individuals can incorporate into their fitness routines.

Optimal bone health is a dynamic interplay between genetics, nutrition, and lifestyle factors. As individuals age, bone density naturally declines, making bones more susceptible to fractures and conditions like osteoporosis. Weight-bearing exercises emerge as a proactive and effective strategy for enhancing bone strength, density, and overall skeletal integrity.

Weight-bearing exercises influence bone remodeling by creating stress on the bones. The mechanical loading induced by these exercises stimulates osteoblast activity, promoting the formation of new bone tissue. This adaptive response leads to increased bone density, strength, and resistance to fractures.

Benefits of Weight-Bearing Exercises for Bone Health:

The benefits of weight-bearing exercises extend beyond the visible improvements in muscle strength and endurance. Specifically, these exercises offer significant advantages for bone health:

1. Increased Bone Density: Weight-bearing exercises, especially those that involve impact and resistance, have been shown to increase bone mineral density. This is particularly important for individuals at risk of osteoporosis or those looking to maintain strong bones as they age.

2. Enhanced Bone Strength: The mechanical stress placed on bones during weight-bearing exercises stimulates the production of collagen and mineralization, contributing to increased bone strength and resilience.

3. Prevention of Bone Loss: Weight-bearing exercises can help counteract age-related bone loss. By engaging in regular strength training, individuals can slow down the rate of bone density decline that typically occurs with aging.

4. Improved Joint Stability: Strong muscles provide support to joints, reducing the risk of falls and fractures. Weight-bearing exercises that target muscles around the joints contribute to improved stability and balance.

5. Enhanced Functional Capacity: Strong bones and muscles contribute to overall functional capacity, allowing individuals to maintain independence and engage in daily activities with ease.

6. Positive Impact on Bone Microarchitecture: Weight-bearing exercises have been shown to positively influence bone microarchitecture, enhancing the trabecular and cortical components of bone tissue. This can contribute to better bone quality and resistance to fractures.

7. Adaptability and Response to Stress: Bones, like muscles, respond to the principle of adaptation. Weight-bearing exercises subject bones to controlled stress, prompting adaptive responses that make them better equipped to handle increased loads.

8. Mitigation of Osteoporosis Risk: Osteoporosis, characterized by low bone mass and deterioration of bone tissue, is a significant concern, especially in postmenopausal women. Weight-bearing exercises serve as a proactive measure to mitigate the risk of osteoporosis.

Types of Weight-Bearing Exercises:

Weight-bearing exercises encompass a broad spectrum of activities, each offering unique benefits for bone health. These exercises can be classified into two main categories: impact and resistance training.

1. Impact Exercises:

 - Impact exercises involve dynamic movements that generate ground reaction forces, stimulating bone adaptation. Examples include:

   - Running and Jogging: High-impact activities like running and jogging subject bones to repeated loading, promoting bone density and strength.

   - Jumping and Plyometrics: Jumping exercises, such as jump squats or box jumps, create rapid and forceful impacts, contributing to bone remodeling.

   - Aerobic Dancing: Dance-based workouts that involve rhythmic and dynamic movements provide a weight-bearing stimulus for bones.

2. Resistance Training:

- Resistance training involves working against an external force, such as weights or resistance bands. It targets specific muscle groups, indirectly benefiting bone health. Examples include:

- Weight Lifting: Using free weights or weight machines to perform exercises like squats, deadlifts, and bench presses engages multiple muscle groups, including those around the bones.

- Bodyweight Exercises: Exercises like push-ups, lunges, and squats use the body's weight as resistance, promoting muscle and bone strength.

- Resistance Bands: These elastic bands provide resistance during exercises, offering a versatile and accessible option for strength training.

Guidelines for Effective Weight-Bearing Exercises:

To maximize the bone health benefits of weight-bearing exercises, it's important to follow guidelines that ensure safety and effectiveness:

1. Gradual Progression: Start with exercises of lower intensity and gradually progress to more challenging activities. This approach allows bones and muscles to adapt to increasing loads over time.

2. Variety of Movements: Incorporate a variety of weight-bearing exercises that target different muscle groups and movement patterns. This ensures comprehensive stimulation of bones throughout the body.

3. Proper Form and Technique: Maintain proper form and technique during exercises to minimize the risk of injury. Consider seeking guidance from fitness professionals or trainers, especially when starting a new exercise program.

4. Individualized Approach: Tailor the intensity and type of weight-bearing exercises based on individual fitness levels, health status, and any pre-existing conditions. Consulting with healthcare providers or fitness professionals can help create personalized exercise plans.

5. Regularity and Consistency: Consistency is key to reaping the benefits of weight-bearing exercises. Aim for regular sessions, incorporating both impact and resistance training, to support ongoing bone remodeling.

6. Consideration of Health Conditions: Individuals with certain health conditions, such as osteoporosis or arthritis, should consult with healthcare providers before engaging in weight-bearing exercises. Modifications and specific recommendations can be made based on individual health needs.

7. Weight-Bearing Activities in Daily Life: Beyond structured exercise sessions, incorporating weight-bearing activities into daily life, such as walking, climbing stairs, or carrying groceries, contributes to cumulative bone-loading effects.

8. Adequate Nutrition: Proper nutrition, including sufficient intake of calcium, vitamin D, and other bone-supportive nutrients, complements the benefits of weight-bearing exercises. A well-balanced diet supports optimal bone remodeling and overall bone health.

9. Monitoring and Adaptation: Periodically reassess exercise routines, considering factors like fitness progression, changes in health status, or evolving fitness goals. Adjustments to the exercise program can be made to ensure continued effectiveness and safety.

10. Cross-Training: Incorporating a variety of physical activities, including aerobic exercises, flexibility training, and balance exercises, complements the benefits of weight-bearing exercises. Cross-training contributes to overall fitness and reduces the risk of overuse injuries.

Challenges and Considerations:

While weight-bearing exercises offer numerous benefits for bone health, certain challenges and considerations should be acknowledged:

1. Age-Related Changes: As individuals age, factors such as decreased bone density, joint stiffness, and muscle weakness may influence the type and intensity of weight-bearing exercises they can safely perform. Tailoring exercise programs to accommodate age-related changes is essential.

2. Joint Health: Individuals with joint conditions, such as arthritis, may need modifications to avoid excessive stress on affected joints. Low-impact variations of weight-bearing exercises or aquatic exercises can be suitable alternatives.

3. Pre-existing Conditions: Certain medical conditions, such as osteoporosis or cardiovascular issues, may require specific considerations when engaging in weight-bearing exercises. Healthcare providers should be consulted to ensure exercise plans align with individual health needs.

4. Accessibility and Resources: Access to fitness facilities, equipment, or professional guidance may vary. Incorporating accessible and cost-effective options, such as walking, bodyweight exercises, or resistance bands, can overcome potential barriers.

5. Motivation and Adherence: Maintaining motivation and adherence to a regular exercise routine can be challenging. Incorporating enjoyable activities, setting realistic goals, and seeking social support can enhance adherence to weight-bearing exercises.

Weight-bearing exercises stand as a cornerstone in the pursuit of optimal bone health. Their impact extends beyond the visible gains in muscle strength, fostering increased bone density, strength, and resilience. Incorporating a variety of impact and resistance training exercises, coupled with proper nutrition and a holistic approach to health, creates a foundation for lifelong bone health. As research continues to unveil the intricacies of bone metabolism and exercise physiology, individuals are empowered to make informed choices that contribute to strong and resilient bones throughout their lives. By embracing weight-bearing exercises as a fundamental component of a healthy lifestyle, individuals can not only prevent bone-related conditions but also enhance their overall physical well-being and quality of life.

CHAPTER SIX

Hormonal Factors and Bone Health

Hormonal factors play a critical role in the intricate dance of maintaining bone health throughout an individual's life. The endocrine system, a network of glands that produce and release hormones, orchestrates various processes, including bone metabolism. Hormones, the chemical messengers of the body, influence bone formation, resorption, and mineralization. In this comprehensive exploration, we delve into the complex interplay between hormones and bone health, examining the roles of key hormones, their effects on bone metabolism, and the implications for overall skeletal well-being.

The skeleton, a dynamic and living tissue, undergoes continuous remodeling throughout life. This remodeling is a finely tuned process of bone resorption and formation, ensuring the maintenance of bone density, strength, and structural integrity. Hormones are integral to this process, exerting profound effects on bone cells and the balance between bone breakdown and formation.

Parathyroid Hormone (PTH):

- Role in Bone Health:

- PTH, produced by the parathyroid glands, plays a central role in calcium homeostasis and bone metabolism.

- When blood calcium levels drop, PTH is released to stimulate the release of calcium from bones, primarily through increased osteoclast activity.

- PTH also enhances the reabsorption of calcium in the kidneys and stimulates the production of active vitamin D, which aids in calcium absorption from the intestines.

- **Clinical Implications:**

- Excessive PTH levels, as seen in conditions like hyperparathyroidism, can lead to increased bone resorption, resulting in weakened bones and a higher risk of fractures.

- Conversely, insufficient PTH levels may contribute to hypocalcemia, impacting bone mineralization.

Calcitonin:

- **Role in Bone Health:**

- Calcitonin, produced by the thyroid gland, opposes the actions of PTH by promoting calcium deposition in bones.

- It inhibits osteoclast activity, reducing bone resorption and helping to regulate blood calcium levels.

- **Clinical Implications:**

- While calcitonin has a regulatory role in calcium metabolism, its impact on overall bone health is less pronounced than that of PTH.

- Calcitonin is sometimes used therapeutically in the management of conditions like osteoporosis.

Vitamin D:

- **Role in Bone Health:**

- Vitamin D is essential for calcium absorption in the intestines, a process crucial for bone mineralization.

- It promotes the differentiation of osteoclasts and osteoblasts, influencing bone remodeling.

- The active form of vitamin D, calcitriol, works in concert with PTH to regulate calcium levels.

- **Clinical Implications:**

- Inadequate vitamin D levels can lead to decreased calcium absorption, contributing to bone disorders like rickets in children and osteomalacia in adults.

- Vitamin D deficiency is associated with an increased risk of fractures and impaired bone health.

Estrogen:

- Role in Bone Health:

- Estrogen, predominantly produced by the ovaries in premenopausal women, has a protective effect on bone density.

- Estrogen inhibits osteoclast activity, reducing bone resorption, and supports the maintenance of bone mass.

- Clinical Implications:

- The decline in estrogen levels during menopause is associated with an accelerated loss of bone density, leading to an increased risk of osteoporosis and fractures.

- Hormone replacement therapy (HRT) may be considered to mitigate bone loss in postmenopausal women, although risks and benefits should be carefully weighed.

Testosterone:

- Role in Bone Health:

- Testosterone, the primary male sex hormone produced by the testes, also contributes to bone health.

- It supports bone formation by stimulating osteoblast activity and has an inhibitory effect on osteoclasts.

- Clinical Implications:

- Low testosterone levels, as observed in conditions like hypogonadism, can lead to decreased bone density and an increased risk of fractures.

- Testosterone replacement therapy may be considered in certain cases to address bone health concerns.

Growth Hormone (GH) and Insulin-Like Growth Factor-1 (IGF-1):

- Role in Bone Health:

- GH, produced by the pituitary gland, stimulates the production of IGF-1 in the liver and other tissues.

- IGF-1 plays a key role in bone growth and development, promoting the proliferation and differentiation of osteoblasts.

- Clinical Implications:

- Deficiencies in GH or IGF-1 during childhood can result in growth retardation and skeletal abnormalities.

- In adulthood, the decline in GH levels is associated with reduced bone density, and GH replacement therapy may be considered in certain cases.

Thyroid Hormones:

- Role in Bone Health:

- Thyroid hormones, including thyroxine (T4) and triiodothyronine (T3), influence bone metabolism.

- Excessive thyroid hormone levels (hyperthyroidism) can lead to increased bone resorption, while insufficient levels (hypothyroidism) may impact bone formation.

- Clinical Implications:

- Hyperthyroidism is associated with an increased risk of osteoporosis and fractures, emphasizing the importance of thyroid function in bone health.

- Maintaining thyroid hormone levels within the normal range is crucial for optimal bone metabolism.

Cortisol:

- Role in Bone Health:

- Cortisol, a steroid hormone produced by the adrenal glands, has complex effects on bone metabolism.

- Prolonged exposure to elevated cortisol levels, as seen in conditions like chronic stress or Cushing's syndrome, can lead to increased bone resorption and decreased bone formation.

- Clinical Implications:

- Chronic glucocorticoid therapy, which mimics the effects of cortisol, is associated with bone loss and an increased risk of fractures. Healthcare providers carefully monitor individuals on long-term glucocorticoid treatment to mitigate these effects.

Insulin:

- Role in Bone Health:

- Insulin, produced by the pancreas, influences bone health through its effects on bone cells and mineralization.

- It plays a role in bone formation and may have an indirect impact on bone density.

- Clinical Implications:

- Conditions associated with insulin resistance, such as type 2 diabetes, may have implications for bone health. Research

is ongoing to understand the complex relationship between insulin and bone metabolism.

Leptin:

- Role in Bone Health:

- Leptin, primarily produced by adipose tissue, influences bone mass through its effects on energy balance.

- It may have both direct and indirect effects on bone cells, modulating bone resorption and formation.

- Clinical Implications:

- Conditions associated with leptin deficiency or resistance, such as certain types of obesity, may have implications for bone health. The relationship between leptin and bone metabolism is an area of active research.

Adiponectin:

- Role in Bone Health:

- Adiponectin, another adipokine produced by adipose tissue, may have implications for bone metabolism.

- Its role in bone health is complex, with some studies suggesting both positive and negative effects on bone density.

   - **Clinical Implications:**

   - The impact of adiponectin on bone health and the potential implications of conditions associated with altered adiponectin levels, such as obesity or metabolic syndrome, are areas of ongoing investigation.

Conclusion:

Hormonal factors intricately govern bone health, influencing the delicate balance between bone formation and resorption. The endocrine system's orchestration of hormones, including PTH, calcitonin, vitamin D, estrogen, testosterone, GH, IGF-1, thyroid hormones, cortisol, insulin, leptin, and adiponectin, shapes the dynamic process of bone remodeling throughout an individual's life. Imbalances in these hormonal factors can contribute to conditions such as osteoporosis, fractures, and metabolic bone disorders. Understanding the roles of hormones in bone health provides insights into preventive and therapeutic strategies, allowing healthcare providers to tailor interventions based on individual hormonal profiles and specific health conditions. As research

continues to unveil the intricacies of hormonal regulation of bone metabolism, the potential for targeted and personalized approaches to optimize bone health emerges, offering hope for improved skeletal well-being and reduced risk of bone-related complications.

CHAPTER SEVEN
Stress Reduction Techniques for Bone Health

Stress, both physical and psychological, can impact various aspects of health, including bone health. Chronic stress has been linked to conditions such as osteoporosis and increased risk of fractures. Recognizing the importance of stress reduction techniques is crucial for maintaining optimal bone health throughout life. In this comprehensive exploration, we delve into the intricate relationship between stress and bone health, examining the physiological mechanisms involved and exploring a diverse range of stress reduction techniques that can positively influence skeletal strength.

The relationship between stress and health is multifaceted, with implications extending to various physiological systems, including the skeletal system. While bones are often associated with structural support and mobility, they are also dynamic tissues that respond to the body's internal and external cues. Chronic stress, whether from physical or psychological sources, can influence bone health through complex mechanisms involving hormones, inflammation, and lifestyle factors. Understanding these connections provides a foundation for exploring effective stress reduction techniques that can contribute to the maintenance of strong and resilient bones.

Physiological Mechanisms:

The impact of stress on bone health involves intricate physiological mechanisms that can influence bone density, remodeling, and susceptibility to fractures. Several key pathways are implicated in this relationship:

1. Hormonal Imbalance:

Chronic stress triggers the release of cortisol, the body's primary stress hormone, from the adrenal glands. Elevated cortisol levels over an extended period can lead to hormonal imbalances, including increased osteoclast activity (cells responsible for bone resorption) and decreased osteoblast activity (cells responsible for bone formation). This imbalance can result in a net loss of bone mass and compromised skeletal integrity.

2. Inflammation:

Stress is associated with increased levels of pro-inflammatory cytokines in the body. Chronic inflammation contributes to bone loss by promoting the activity of osteoclasts and inhibiting

osteoblast function. Inflammatory processes can disrupt the delicate balance of bone remodeling, potentially leading to conditions such as osteoporosis.

3. Lifestyle Factors:

High-stress levels are often linked to unhealthy lifestyle choices, such as poor dietary habits, lack of physical activity, and disruptions in sleep patterns. These factors can independently impact bone health and, when combined with stress, create a cumulative effect that may contribute to bone-related complications.

Stress Reduction Techniques:

Recognizing the interconnectedness of stress and bone health highlights the importance of implementing stress reduction techniques as part of a holistic approach to well-being. Various practices and strategies have demonstrated efficacy in mitigating the physiological effects of stress and promoting overall health, including skeletal strength.

1. Mindfulness Meditation:

Mindfulness meditation involves cultivating present-moment awareness and non-judgmental acceptance. Practices such as mindfulness-based stress reduction (MBSR) have been shown to reduce cortisol levels and improve psychological well-being. Incorporating mindfulness into daily routines can create a positive impact on both mental and physical aspects of health.

2. Yoga:

Yoga combines physical postures, breath control, and meditation to promote relaxation and stress reduction. Regular yoga practice has been associated with lower cortisol levels and improved mood. Weight-bearing yoga poses can also contribute to bone health by promoting muscle strength and balance.

3. Deep Breathing Exercises:

Deep breathing exercises, such as diaphragmatic breathing or pranayama, activate the body's relaxation response. By slowing down the breath and promoting diaphragmatic engagement, these techniques help reduce stress hormones, enhance oxygenation, and create a sense of calm.

4. Progressive Muscle Relaxation (PMR):

PMR involves systematically tensing and then relaxing different muscle groups to promote physical and mental relaxation. This technique can alleviate muscle tension, reduce stress, and contribute to an overall sense of well-being.

5. Tai Chi:

Tai Chi is a mind-body practice that combines gentle movements with deep breathing and mindfulness. Studies suggest that Tai Chi can reduce cortisol levels, improve balance, and positively impact bone density, particularly in older adults.

6. Biofeedback:

Biofeedback is a technique that allows individuals to monitor and control physiological responses, such as heart rate and muscle tension, with the help of electronic devices. Learning to regulate these responses can promote relaxation and reduce the physiological impact of stress on the body.

7. Guided Imagery:

Guided imagery involves using the imagination to create calming and positive mental images. This technique can help shift focus away from stressors, promote relaxation, and contribute to a more positive emotional state.

8. Physical Activity and Exercise:

Regular physical activity has dual benefits for bone health and stress reduction. Weight-bearing exercises, such as walking, jogging, or resistance training, contribute to bone density, while the release of endorphins during exercise promotes a sense of well-being and reduces stress.

9. Social Support:

Building and maintaining strong social connections can provide a valuable buffer against stress. Engaging in activities with friends and family, sharing experiences, and receiving emotional support contribute to a sense of belonging and resilience in the face of stressors.

10. Adequate Sleep:

Quality sleep is essential for overall health, including bone health. Chronic stress can disrupt sleep patterns, and conversely, insufficient sleep can exacerbate stress. Establishing a consistent sleep routine and creating a conducive sleep environment can positively impact both stress and bone health.

Implementation and Integration:

Incorporating stress reduction techniques into daily life requires a proactive and individualized approach. The effectiveness of these techniques often lies in their regular practice and integration into one's lifestyle. Creating a personalized stress reduction plan may involve a combination of different techniques based on individual preferences and needs.

1. Establishing Routine:

Consistency is key when implementing stress reduction techniques. Establishing a daily or weekly routine that includes designated times for practices such as meditation, yoga, or exercise helps make these activities a regular part of life.

2. Experimenting with Techniques:

Individuals may resonate differently with various stress reduction techniques. Experimenting with different practices allows for the identification of those that align with personal preferences and provide the most significant benefit.

3. Combining Strategies:

Combining multiple stress reduction strategies can enhance their overall impact. For example, pairing mindfulness meditation with regular physical activity creates a synergistic effect that addresses both psychological and physiological aspects of stress.

4. Seeking Professional Guidance:

For individuals dealing with chronic stress or specific health concerns, seeking guidance from healthcare professionals, psychologists, or certified instructors can provide tailored strategies and support.

Stress reduction is a vital component of maintaining optimal bone health and overall well-being. The intricate relationship between stress and physiological processes, including those affecting bone metabolism, underscores the importance of addressing stress as part of a comprehensive health strategy. Implementing stress reduction techniques, whether through mindfulness practices, physical activity, or social support, can contribute to a positive impact on bone density, remodeling, and resilience. By recognizing the interconnectedness of mental and physical health, individuals can empower themselves to proactively manage stress and foster skeletal strength throughout their lives. As research continues to uncover the nuances of stress and its effects on the body, the integration of evidence-based stress reduction techniques becomes increasingly valuable in promoting holistic health and enhancing the quality of life.

CHAPTER EIGHT

Sleep and Its Role in Bone Regeneration

Sleep is a fundamental aspect of human physiology that plays a critical role in overall health and well-being. Beyond its well-established impact on mental function and emotional regulation, sleep has profound effects on various physiological processes, including bone regeneration. In this comprehensive exploration, we delve into the intricate relationship between sleep and bone health, examining the mechanisms through which sleep influences bone regeneration, the consequences of insufficient sleep, and strategies for optimizing sleep to support robust skeletal function.

The importance of sleep for human health is undeniable, with a myriad of physiological functions influenced by the quality and duration of sleep. One area that has garnered increasing attention in research is the relationship between sleep and bone health. Bones are dynamic tissues undergoing constant remodeling, a process that involves the delicate balance between bone resorption and formation. Sleep is emerging as a crucial factor in supporting the regenerative aspects of this process, influencing bone mineral density, strength, and overall skeletal integrity.

Mechanisms of Sleep and Bone Interaction:

The interplay between sleep and bone regeneration involves intricate physiological mechanisms that occur during different stages of sleep. Understanding these mechanisms provides insights into the ways in which sleep influences bone health.

1. Growth Hormone Release:

During deep sleep, particularly during the slow-wave sleep (SWS) stage, the pituitary gland releases growth hormone (GH). GH is a key player in bone health, stimulating the production of insulin-like growth factor-1 (IGF-1), which, in turn, promotes bone growth and regeneration. Insufficient sleep, especially a lack of deep sleep, can compromise the release of GH and impact bone health.

2. Melatonin Production:

Melatonin, often referred to as the "sleep hormone," is produced by the pineal gland, and its levels rise during the evening and night. Melatonin has been shown to have protective effects on bone health by modulating bone metabolism, reducing oxidative stress, and influencing the activity of bone-forming cells (osteoblasts). Disruptions in the natural circadian rhythm, such as those caused

by irregular sleep patterns or exposure to artificial light at night, can affect melatonin production and potentially impact bone regeneration.

3. Circadian Rhythms and Bone Turnover:

The circadian rhythm, the body's internal clock, regulates various physiological processes, including bone turnover. Bone resorption and formation exhibit circadian variations, with increased bone resorption during the night and increased bone formation during the day. Disruptions to circadian rhythms, such as those associated with shift work or irregular sleep schedules, can disrupt this balance and affect bone health.

4. Inflammatory Modulation:

Adequate sleep is associated with the regulation of inflammatory processes in the body. Chronic inflammation is linked to increased bone resorption and decreased bone formation, contributing to conditions like osteoporosis. Sleep deprivation or poor sleep quality may exacerbate inflammation, negatively impacting bone health.

Consequences of Insufficient Sleep on Bone Health:

Insufficient or poor-quality sleep can have detrimental effects on bone health, potentially contributing to the development of skeletal disorders and increasing the risk of fractures. Several consequences highlight the significance of prioritizing adequate and restorative sleep for optimal bone regeneration.

1. Reduced Growth Hormone Secretion:

Insufficient sleep, particularly a lack of deep sleep, can impair the release of growth hormone. This reduction in growth hormone secretion diminishes the stimulation of IGF-1, which plays a pivotal role in bone growth and repair. As a result, bone regeneration may be compromised, potentially leading to decreased bone density and strength.

2. Altered Circadian Rhythms:

Irregular sleep patterns, such as those associated with shift work or inconsistent sleep schedules, can disrupt circadian rhythms. This disruption may lead to an imbalance in bone turnover, with consequences for both bone resorption and formation. The long-term impact of circadian misalignment on bone health underscores the importance of maintaining consistent sleep-wake cycles.

3. Increased Inflammatory Markers:

Inadequate sleep is associated with an increase in inflammatory markers in the body. Elevated inflammation contributes to bone resorption and inhibits bone formation, potentially accelerating the progression of conditions like osteoporosis. Chronic exposure to inflammation due to poor sleep may create an unfavorable environment for optimal bone health.

4. Impaired Immune Function:

Sleep is intricately connected to immune function, and inadequate sleep can compromise the body's ability to mount an effective immune response. Impaired immune function may contribute to chronic low-grade inflammation, negatively influencing bone health and regeneration.

Optimizing Sleep for Bone Regeneration:

Recognizing the importance of sleep in supporting bone regeneration emphasizes the need to prioritize healthy sleep habits. Implementing strategies to optimize sleep quality and duration contributes not only to skeletal health but also to overall well-being.

1. Establishing a Consistent Sleep Schedule:

Going to bed and waking up at the same time each day helps regulate the circadian rhythm and supports the natural sleep-wake cycle. Consistency in sleep schedules enhances the body's ability to synchronize physiological processes, including bone turnover.

2. Creating a Relaxing Bedtime Routine:

Engaging in calming activities before bedtime signals to the body that it is time to wind down. Establishing a relaxing bedtime routine, such as reading, gentle stretching, or practicing relaxation techniques, promotes a smoother transition into restful sleep.

3. Optimizing Sleep Environment:

Creating a conducive sleep environment involves considerations such as maintaining a cool and dark room, investing in a comfortable mattress and pillows, and minimizing noise and light disruptions. An optimal sleep environment enhances the quality of sleep and its potential impact on bone regeneration.

4. Limiting Exposure to Artificial Light:

Exposure to artificial light, especially the blue light emitted by screens, can suppress melatonin production and disrupt circadian rhythms. Limiting screen time before bedtime and using blue light filters on electronic devices contribute to a more natural sleep-wake cycle.

5. Regular Physical Activity:

Regular physical activity has been associated with improved sleep quality. Engaging in moderate-intensity exercise, such as walking or cycling, promotes better sleep patterns and contributes to overall health, including bone health.

6. Managing Stress and Anxiety:

Stress and anxiety can interfere with the ability to fall asleep and maintain restful sleep. Implementing stress reduction techniques, such as mindfulness meditation or deep breathing exercises, can help manage stress and create a more relaxed bedtime environment.

7. Avoiding Stimulants Before Bed:

Stimulants such as caffeine and nicotine can interfere with sleep. Avoiding the consumption of stimulants in the hours leading up to bedtime supports the body's natural sleep processes.

8. Seeking Professional Guidance:

Individuals experiencing persistent sleep disturbances or sleep disorders may benefit from seeking guidance from healthcare professionals, such as sleep specialists or physicians. Addressing underlying sleep-related issues can contribute to improved bone health.

The intricate relationship between sleep and bone regeneration highlights the essential role of adequate and restorative sleep in maintaining optimal skeletal health. The physiological mechanisms connecting sleep to bone metabolism underscore the significance of prioritizing healthy sleep habits as a fundamental aspect of a holistic approach to well-being. As research continues to unveil the complexities of sleep's influence on bone health, individuals are empowered to make informed choices that support both the quantity and quality of their sleep. By recognizing sleep as a pillar of overall health, individuals can enhance the regenerative capacity of their bones, promoting resilience and strength throughout the lifespan.

CHAPTER NINE

Monitoring and Assessing Bone Density

Monitoring and assessing bone density is a critical component of preventive healthcare, particularly in the context of conditions such as osteoporosis and osteopenia. Bones provide structural support to the body, and their density is indicative of their strength and resilience. Various methods and technologies are employed to measure bone density, helping healthcare professionals identify individuals at risk of fractures and design appropriate interventions. In this comprehensive exploration, we delve into the importance of monitoring bone density, the techniques used for assessment, and the implications for overall bone health.

Bone density is a key parameter in evaluating the health and strength of the skeletal system. The density of bones reflects the amount of mineral content, primarily calcium and phosphorus, within the bone tissue. Monitoring bone density is crucial for identifying conditions such as osteoporosis, a systemic skeletal disorder characterized by low bone mass and deterioration of bone tissue, leading to an increased risk of fractures.

Importance of Monitoring Bone Density:

Monitoring bone density serves several important purposes in the realm of healthcare and preventive medicine. Understanding the significance of this process is foundational to appreciating its role in maintaining optimal bone health.

1. Early Detection of Osteoporosis:

Osteoporosis often develops silently, with no noticeable symptoms until a fracture occurs. Monitoring bone density enables early detection of reduced bone mass, allowing healthcare professionals to intervene before fractures occur. Early detection is key to implementing preventive measures and minimizing the impact of osteoporosis.

2. Fracture Risk Assessment:

Low bone density is a major contributor to fractures, especially in weight-bearing bones such as the hip, spine, and wrist. Assessing bone density provides valuable information for estimating an individual's risk of fractures. This risk assessment guides healthcare providers in tailoring interventions to reduce the likelihood of fractures.

3. Evaluation of Treatment Efficacy:

For individuals undergoing treatment for osteoporosis or related bone disorders, monitoring bone density allows healthcare professionals to assess the effectiveness of therapeutic interventions. Changes in bone density over time provide insights into the success of treatment regimens and help adjust strategies as needed.

4. Identification of High-Risk Populations:

Certain populations are more prone to low bone density and osteoporosis. Monitoring bone density aids in identifying high-risk groups, such as postmenopausal women and older adults, allowing for targeted screening and interventions. This proactive approach is essential for preventing fractures and associated complications.

Techniques for Assessing Bone Density:

Several techniques and technologies are employed to assess bone density, each with its advantages and limitations. These methods provide quantitative data on bone density and assist healthcare professionals in making informed decisions regarding patient care.

1. Dual-Energy X-ray Absorptiometry (DXA):

DXA is the gold standard for measuring bone density. It uses low-dose X-rays to assess bone mineral content and density at specific skeletal sites, typically the hip and spine. DXA results are reported as T-scores, comparing an individual's bone density to that of a healthy young adult. A T-score of -1 and above is considered normal, while scores between -1 and -2.5 indicate osteopenia, and scores below -2.5 suggest osteoporosis.

2. Quantitative Computed Tomography (QCT):

QCT utilizes computed tomography (CT) scans to measure bone mineral density. Unlike DXA, QCT provides three-dimensional images and can assess bone density in specific regions of interest. QCT is particularly useful for evaluating trabecular and cortical bone separately. It is commonly used in research settings and may be employed when DXA results are inconclusive.

3. Peripheral Dual-Energy X-ray Absorptiometry (pDXA):

Similar to DXA, pDXA assesses bone density at peripheral sites, such as the forearm or heel. While not as precise as central DXA, pDXA is a portable and more accessible option for screening and monitoring bone density at the periphery. It is often used in community settings and mobile clinics.

4. Quantitative Ultrasound (QUS):

QUS measures bone density using high-frequency sound waves. This non-invasive technique is often employed to assess bone density in peripheral sites, such as the heel or finger. QUS provides an estimate of bone mineral density and has the advantage of being radiation-free. However, it may not be as accurate as DXA in certain populations.

5. Magnetic Resonance Imaging (MRI):

MRI, primarily used for soft tissue imaging, can also provide information about bone density. While not as commonly employed as DXA or QCT for bone density assessment, MRI is valuable in specific clinical scenarios, such as evaluating bone marrow composition and detecting abnormalities in bone structure.

6. Biochemical Markers of Bone Turnover:

Blood tests measuring specific markers of bone turnover, such as serum calcium, phosphorus, and bone-specific alkaline phosphatase, can provide indirect information about bone health. While these markers are not direct measures of bone density, they offer insights into bone metabolism and turnover.

Interpretation of Bone Density Results:

Interpreting bone density results requires an understanding of the reference values, the specific technique used, and the patient's individual characteristics. Healthcare professionals consider various factors to make informed decisions based on bone density assessments.

1. T-Scores and Z-Scores:

 T-scores compare an individual's bone density to that of a healthy young adult, while Z-scores compare bone density to an age-matched peer group. T-scores are commonly used in diagnosing osteoporosis and osteopenia. A lower T-score indicates lower bone density relative to the reference population.

2. Diagnostic Categories:

Based on T-scores, bone density results are categorized into diagnostic groups:

- Normal: T-score of -1.0 and above.

- Osteopenia: T-score between -1.0 and -2.5.

- Osteoporosis: T-score of -2.5 and below.

3. Clinical Risk Factors:

Healthcare professionals consider clinical risk factors when interpreting bone density results. Factors such as age, sex, family history of fractures, and the presence of other medical conditions influence fracture risk and guide decision-making regarding treatment and preventive measures.

4. Trend Analysis:

Monitoring changes in bone density over time is essential for assessing treatment efficacy and disease progression. Trend analysis involves comparing sequential bone density measurements to identify stability, improvement, or decline in bone health.

Implications for Overall Bone Health:

Assessing and monitoring bone density contribute to a comprehensive understanding of overall bone health. Beyond diagnosing osteoporosis, bone density results inform healthcare providers about an individual's risk of fractures and guide interventions to optimize skeletal strength.

1. Individualized Treatment Plans:

Bone density results play a pivotal role in developing individualized treatment plans. For individuals with osteopenia or osteoporosis, healthcare professionals may recommend lifestyle modifications, pharmacological interventions, and specific exercises to enhance bone health.

2. Lifestyle Modifications:

Individuals with low bone density are often advised to incorporate lifestyle modifications that support bone health. These may include a diet rich in calcium and vitamin D, weight-bearing exercises, smoking cessation, and limiting alcohol intake. Monitoring bone density allows for adjustments to these recommendations based on individual needs.

3. Pharmacological Interventions:

In cases of osteoporosis or high fracture risk, pharmacological interventions may be recommended. Medications such as bisphosphonates, denosumab, or hormone replacement therapy aim to reduce bone resorption and enhance bone density. Monitoring bone density helps assess the effectiveness of these interventions and guides treatment decisions.

4. Fall Prevention Strategies:

Low bone density increases the risk of fractures, especially in the context of falls. Monitoring bone density is crucial for identifying individuals at risk and implementing fall prevention strategies. These may include balance exercises, home modifications, and vision assessments to reduce the likelihood of falls and fractures.

5. Patient Education and Empowerment:

Understanding one's bone density results empowers individuals to actively participate in their bone health. Patient education regarding the implications of bone density, lifestyle factors influencing bone health, and the role of preventive measures fosters a proactive approach to skeletal well-being.

Monitoring and assessing bone density are integral components of preventive healthcare, providing valuable insights into skeletal strength and fracture risk. The diverse techniques available for bone density assessment offer healthcare professionals options to tailor diagnostic approaches based on individual needs and clinical scenarios. Beyond the diagnosis of osteoporosis, bone density results guide the development of personalized treatment plans, lifestyle modifications, and interventions to optimize overall bone health. As research continues to advance in the field of bone health, the integration of innovative technologies and a holistic understanding

of skeletal physiology contribute to enhanced preventive strategies and improved outcomes for individuals at risk of bone-related complications.

CONCLUSION
Taking Charge of Your Bone Health

In the journey towards optimal well-being, the proactive management of bone health emerges as a pivotal aspect of overall health. As we've navigated the intricate landscape of bone health, from understanding the complexities of osteoporosis and osteopenia to exploring evidence-based interventions and lifestyle modifications, one resounding theme remains: the power of individual agency in taking charge of one's bone health.

Empowerment through Knowledge:

Knowledge is a potent tool in the pursuit of health, and in the realm of bone health, understanding the nuances of osteoporosis, osteopenia, and the factors influencing skeletal strength is the first step towards empowerment. Armed with knowledge, individuals gain the capacity to make informed decisions about their lifestyles, habits, and healthcare choices. It is the foundation upon which the proactive journey towards robust bone health is built.

Lifestyle as a Cornerstone:

The choices we make in our daily lives reverberate through the health of our bones. From the foods we consume to the physical activities we engage in, lifestyle choices play a fundamental role in shaping bone density and resilience. The incorporation of a balanced diet rich in calcium and vitamin D, coupled with weight-bearing exercises and the avoidance of detrimental habits like smoking and excessive alcohol consumption, sets the stage for fortified skeletal strength.

Preventive Measures as Safeguards:

Prevention is a powerful strategy in the realm of bone health. By adopting preventive measures, individuals can mitigate the risk of bone-related complications and fractures. Regular health check-ups, screenings for bone density, and adherence to evidence-based interventions contribute to a proactive approach that safeguards against the insidious onset of conditions like osteoporosis.

Holistic Wellness:

Taking charge of bone health extends beyond the confines of bone density measurements and pharmacological interventions. It embraces a holistic approach to wellness that encompasses mental, emotional, and physical dimensions. Stress reduction techniques, adequate sleep, and mindfulness practices not only fortify bones indirectly but also contribute to overall well-being. Recognizing the interconnectedness of various aspects of health empowers individuals to foster a harmonious balance that radiates through their entire being.

The Role of Healthcare Professionals:

In this journey towards taking charge of bone health, the partnership between individuals and healthcare professionals is integral. Regular consultations, open communication, and collaborative decision-making create a synergy that amplifies the effectiveness of interventions. Healthcare providers serve as guides, offering personalized insights and evidence-based recommendations that empower individuals to make choices aligned with their unique health needs.

A Lifelong Commitment:

Taking charge of bone health is not a fleeting endeavor but a lifelong commitment to well-being. As individuals progress through different life stages, from adolescence to adulthood and into the golden years, the strategies for optimizing bone health may evolve. It requires adaptability, a willingness to embrace new information, and a commitment to prioritizing health as an ongoing journey rather than a destination.

In conclusion, taking charge of your bone health is a profound act of self-care and resilience. It is an acknowledgment of the remarkable capabilities of the human body and a commitment to nurturing its foundational structure—the skeletal system. By integrating knowledge, adopting a lifestyle that nurtures bone health, engaging in preventive measures, and fostering a holistic approach to wellness, individuals can embark on a journey that transcends the prevention of bone-related complications—it is a journey towards a vibrant, active, and fulfilling life.

In this journey, every choice matters. Every step towards a nutritious meal, every moment spent in physical activity, every decision to prioritize sleep, and every instance of stress reduction becomes a testament to the commitment to bone health. It is a journey not just for today but for the years to come—an investment in a future where the skeletal system stands as a resilient pillar supporting a life well-lived.

So, take charge—embrace the knowledge, make informed choices, and cultivate habits that resonate with the vitality of your bones. In doing so, you not only fortify the structural integrity of your body but also pave the way for a life of strength, flexibility, and enduring well-being. Your

bones are the silent architects of your movement, and by taking charge, you become the steward of their enduring strength.

www.ingramcontent.com/pod-product-compliance
Lightning Source LLC
Chambersburg PA
CBHW080726260726
48660CB00010B/3713